Understanding and Treating Borderline Personality Disorder

A Guide for Professionals and Families

Understanding and Treating Borderline Personality Disorder

A Guide for Professionals and Families

Edited by

John G. Gunderson, M.D.

Perry D. Hoffman, Ph.D.

In Collaboration With

Penny Steiner-Grossman, Ed.D., M.P.H.

Patricia Woodward, M.A.T.

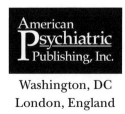

Washington, DC
London, England

Copyright © 2005 American Psychiatric Publishing, Inc.
ALL RIGHTS RESERVED

Manufactured in the United States of America on acid-free paper
09   08   07   06   05   5   4   3   2
First Edition

Typeset in Adobe's New Baskerville and Optima/Optima ExtraBlack

American Psychiatric Publishing, Inc.
1000 Wilson Boulevard
Arlington, VA 22209-3901
www.appi.org

Library of Congress Cataloging-in-Publication Data
Understanding and treating borderline personality disorder : a guide
   for professionals and families / edited by John G. Gunderson,
   Perry D. Hoffman ; in collaboration with Penny Steiner-Grossman,
   Patricia Woodward. – 1st ed.
      p. ; cm.
   Includes bibliographical references and index.
   ISBN 1-58562-135-8 (pbk. : alk. paper)
   1. Borderline personality disorder. 2. Borderline personality
disorder–Treatment. 3. Borderline personality disorder–Patients
–Family relationships.   I. Gunderson, John G., 1942-   .
II. Hoffman, Perry D., 1944-   .
   [DNLM: 1. Borderline Personality Disorder. 2. Family Health.
3. Professional-Family Relations.   WM 190 U545 2005]
RC569.5.B67U53 2005
616.85'852–dc22
                              2004027569

British Library Cataloguing in Publication Data
A CIP record is available from the British Library.

Contents

Part I
Diagnosis, Treatment,
and Prognosis

Part II
Family Matters

Contributors

C. Christian Beels, M.D., M.S.
Former Director, Public Psychiatry Fellowship, New York State Psychiatric Institute, New York, New York

Donna S. Bender, Ph.D.
Assistant Clinical Professor of Medical Psychology in Psychiatry, Columbia University College of Physicians and Surgeons; Research Scientist, Department of Personality Studies, New York State Psychiatric Institute, New York, New York

Jennifer L. Boulanger, B.A.
Doctoral student, Department of Psychology, University of Nevada, Reno, Nevada

Beth S. Brodsky, Ph.D.
Research Scientist, Department of Neuroscience, New York State Psychiatric Institute; Department of Psychiatry, Columbia University College of Physicians and Surgeons, New York, New York

Alan E. Fruzzetti, Ph.D.
Associate Professor of Psychology; Director, Dialectical Behavior Therapy and Research Program, University of Nevada, Reno, Nevada

John G. Gunderson, M.D.
Director, Center for Treatment and Research on Borderline Personality Disorder, McLean Hospital, Belmont, Massachusetts; Professor in Psychiatry, Harvard Medical School, Boston, Massachusetts

Perry D. Hoffman, Ph.D.
President, National Education Alliance for Borderline Personality Disorder; Research Associate, Weill Medical College, Cornell University, New York, New York

Harriet P. Lefley, Ph.D.
Professor of Psychiatry and Behavioral Sciences, University of Miami School of Medicine, Miami, Florida

John M. Oldham, M.D.
Professor and Chairman, Department of Psychiatry and Behavioral Sciences; Executive Director, Institute of Psychiatry, Medical University of South Carolina, Charleston, South Carolina

Dixianne Penney, Dr.P.H.
Executive Vice President, National Education Alliance for Borderline Personality Disorder, Rye, New York; Administrative Director, Center for the Study of Issues in Public Mental Health, Orangeburg, New York

Andrew E. Skodol, M.D.
Professor of Clinical Psychiatry, Columbia University College of Physicians and Surgeons; Director, Department of Personality Studies, New York State Psychiatric Institute, New York, New York

Paul H. Soloff, M.D.
Professor of Psychiatry, Western Psychiatric Institute and Clinic, University of Pittsburgh Medical School, Pittsburgh, Pennsylvania

Barbara Stanley, Ph.D.
Research Scientist, Department of Neuroscience, New York State Psychiatric Institute, Columbia University College of Physicians and Surgeons; Professor of Psychology, City University of New York–John Jay College, New York, New York

Penny Steiner-Grossman, Ed.D.
Assistant Dean for Educational Resources and Associate Professor of Clinical Family and Social Medicine, Albert Einstein College of Medicine of Yeshiva University, Bronx, New York

Patricia Woodward, M.A.T.
Secretary, National Education Alliance for Borderline Personality Disorder, Rye, New York

Mary C. Zanarini, Ed.D.
Associate Professor of Psychology and Director, Laboratory for the Study of Adult Development, Harvard Medical School, Boston, Massachusetts

Foreword

An attractive professional woman was meeting with me to discuss the possibility of psychotherapy for herself. I had recently finished seeing her and her ex-husband (a therapist) to deal with some of the unfinished business of their separation, and now she and I were talking about what kind of further consultation might benefit her.

"Fortunately," I said, "there are new and really effective forms of therapies that will help you—one specifically designed for your kind of problem."

"Oh," she said, "What kind of problem is that?"

Realizing I had drifted into an area of unknown danger, I tried to skirt it. "The name is really not so important as the fact that there are some good ideas about how to work with it."

"But is it a diagnosis?" she persisted—"I've always wondered if these difficulties that keep happening to me have a name.'

"They're called borderline problems," I said, offhandedly, "but the treatment is called…" Her face froze at the word. "Oh, no," she said, "I know what 'borderline' means—infuriating, demanding. I remember the parties where my ex-husband and his colleagues joked about their borderline patients, about how awful and how impossible they are. If that's what all of you think I am, no wonder I've always had so much trouble getting anything out of therapy." She gathered her belongings together and prepared to leave my office. Nothing I could say would induce her to stay and hear the good news—that when the diagnosis is made central to treatment, the therapies often go well. It's when the diagnosis is overlooked that it is hard to get anything out of therapy. She had seen this diagnostic label from the inside, professional point of view, and she fled from it.

As I thought about this scene afterward, I realized it highlighted the difference between two approaches, or eras, in the treatment of borderline personality disorder (BPD). In the first era, from the 1940s until rather recently—and clearly, for some, such as this woman's ex-husband, extending into the present—the mention of BPD provoked a kind of special dread. Many believe it can be treated only by some very hardy, talented people with a special temperament for the work. One of my teachers in residency (1961–1964) said it was "like trying to do therapy with a startled faun." Those of us unable to take the strain of trying over months and years to get close enough to earn the trust of such difficult people excused ourselves. We told war stories about how we had been ambushed by referrals that had not warned us of this diagnosis. We advised each other not to have more than one such patient in our practice at any one time. "She will use up all your spare supervision resources and the patience of your colleagues who don't want to hear about it, to say nothing of your sleep and your self-esteem as an effective therapist."

This was the era of solo psychoanalytic therapy, when indeed little was taught about the treatment except that it was extremely difficult and demanding. But wasn't it difficult and demanding partly because we were expecting it to be like the psychotherapy we were conducting with our neurotic, "worried well" patients? It had not occurred to us that we were part of the problem, making it more difficult for ourselves and our patients by insisting on the same psychoanalytic assumptions, modified by our ideas about "the borderline transference." This was the blame-the-victim idea that BPD patients always make exaggerated demands of their therapists and thus always encounter correspondingly exaggerated disappointment. These dilemmas and their more modern solutions are well described by Donna S. Bender, Ph.D., and John M. Oldham, M.D., in Chapter 2 of this volume, "Psychotherapies for Borderline Personality Disorder."

In the 1990s all of this began to change with the arrival of a new climate of research and therapy, in which this book takes part. In this new era, several things have changed:

1. Epidemiological research (reviewed by Andrew E. Skodol, M.D., in Chapter 1, "The Borderline Diagnosis: Concepts, Criteria, and Controversies," with a review of the research by Mary C. Zanarini, Ed.D., in Chapter 5, "The Longitudinal Course of Borderline Personality Disorder"), in which it was clear that the illness could have an improving course. One study that had a particular impact was the long-term follow-up by Stone (1990) of a large number of patients many years after they had left the inpatient treatment program at the New York State Psychiatric Institute. He discovered that it was not unusual for patients to leave therapy for periods of time and that it was therefore not disgraceful or a sign of failure on the part of either the patient or the therapist. Many patients who went from therapist to therapist got

better. And some whose personal lives were terribly disappointing nevertheless managed to learn self-esteem in the world of work, and this helped them later in life.

2. Pharmacology research (described by Paul H. Soloff, M.D., in Chapter 4, "Pharmacotherapy in Borderline Personality Disorder") that has discovered that some patients are helped by medication. This development had both the direct effect of providing benefit from the medication and the indirect effect of validating the condition as a treatable vulnerability of the nervous system rather than as a failure of "character." To the lay reader, the fact that in earlier literature "borderline" was listed as a "character" disorder made it seem even more repellant.

3. New understanding, as shown in Judith Herman's highly readable and popular book *Trauma and Recovery* (Herman 1992), put BPD in the context of a variety of conditions related to traumatic experiences, such as combat fatigue and multiple personality disorder. The public's interest in the phenomenon of trauma and its treatment produced a different, sympathetic atmosphere that overflowed into the popular press with the World Trade Center disaster.

4. New treatments such as dialectical behavior therapy (DBT) (Linehan et al. 1994) emphasized that neither therapists nor patients were alone in their struggles with this problem and that indeed it could be objectified and described in a way that highlighted its cognitive-behavioral aspects. Social sequences and cues to interpersonal misunderstanding could be discussed in groups of people who had all had similar experiences, and this public airing put the emotions of fear, resentment, and disappointment into an objective frame from which something could be learned. Linehan's successful program of disseminating her methods had a major impact on professionals, who began to see that DBT could be learned and that work with BPD did not require sainthood or genius.

Understanding and Treating Borderline Personality Disorder: A Guide for Professionals and Families now furthers the development of this new era of treatment by bringing in the missing element in the picture, the perspectives of consumers and families, presented here in the following chapters: Chapter 6, "Living with Borderline Personality Disorder: Two Firsthand Accounts"; Chapter 7, "Family Perspectives on Borderline Personality Disorder," by Dixianne Penney, Dr.P.H., and Patricia Woodward, M.A.T; Chapter 8, "From Family Trauma to Family Support System," by Harriet P. Lefley, Ph.D.; and Chapter 9, "Family Involvement in Treatment," by Alan E. Fruzzetti, Ph.D., and Jennifer L. Boulanger, B.A.

• • •

Until now, therapists have lacked ways in which to educate both family and patient to see themselves as victimized by the illness. So they have set up a private, "neutral" relationship with the patient that, on the psychoanalytic model, excludes and ignores the family.

• • •

Families have been missing from the plan for a number of reasons, which Dr. Lefley reviews in her discussion of the sources of the painful ambiguity and difficulty of their position. Therapists have not wanted to "negotiate between the dangerous shoals of blaming the family and blaming the patient." Until now, they have lacked a way of educating both family and patient to see themselves as victimized by the illness, and so they have set up a private, "neutral" relationship with the patient that, on the psychoanalytic model, excludes and ignores the family. Conversely, patients have tended to stay away from conferences and multifamily groups organized for their family members (Berkowitz and Gunderson 2002). This book begins to explore the basis for common ground in a new, no-blame way of understanding the illness and its treatment.

In addition to the chapters mentioned so far, I would call attention to Chapter 3 by Barbara Stanley, Ph.D., and Beth S. Brodsky, Ph.D., "Suicidal and Self-Injurious Behavior in Borderline Personality Disorder: A Self-Regulation Model." This chapter presents in detail the subjective experience, neurophysiology, and clinical interaction that accompany the most distressing feature of BPD, the tendency to engage in self-harm. I think reading and discussion of this chapter—perhaps even a discussion involving patients, family members, and therapists together—could provide a way of talking together about specific experiences.

In sum, *Understanding and Treating Borderline Personality Disorder: A Guide for Professionals and Families* is a helpful, practical book in an area of pain and suffering that is now beginning to emerge into the light of shared knowledge. With it, BPD begins to take its place with other distinctive emotional disorders, as a barrier to be overcome or a handicap to be lived with rather than a sentence to despair.

C. Christian Beels, M.D., M.S.

References

Berkowitz CB, Gunderson JG: Multifamily psychoeducational treatment of borderline personality disorder, in The Multifamily Group. Edited by McFarlane WR. New York, Oxford University Press, 2002, pp 258–290

Herman JL: Trauma and Recovery. New York, Basic Books, 1992

Linehan MM, Tutek DA, Heard HL, et al: Interpersonal outcome of cognitive behavioral treatment for chronically suicidal borderline patients. Am J Psychiatry 151:1771–1776, 1994

Stone M: The Fate of Borderline Patients: Successful Outcome and Psychiatric Practice. New York, Guilford, 1990

Preface

Often devastating, borderline personality disorder (BPD) is an illness that not only affects individuals with the diagnosis but also intensely affects those who care about them. The goal of *Understanding and Treating Borderline Personality Disorder: A Guide for Professionals and Families* is to provide information and education to reduce the confusion and isolation that typically accompany this disorder.

● ● ●

> More than a decade ago, we became concerned that the mental health field had failed to recognize the family's perspective on BPD. These families were troubled by the same problems that vexed mental health professionals—problems that are even more deeply demoralizing for families.

● ● ●

The direct inspiration for this book came from the first annual conference of the National Education Alliance for Borderline Personality Disorder (NEA-BPD). That conference, entitled "From Research to Community: Family Perspectives on Borderline Personality Disorder," was held in New York in October 2002. At the conference, most of this book's chapter authors (family members, consumers, and professionals) made presentations in their areas of experience. The more than 400 who attended included family members who had been affected by this disorder and an impressive number of mental health professionals who wanted to learn more about it. Many who could not attend the conference asked us to share the information in the presentations. We are extremely grateful to all our chapter authors for taking the time to adapt their presentations or their writings. Together these chapters reflect wide-ranging and updated perspectives on BPD that ensure the book's goal will be fulfilled for readers.

Nearly a decade before the NEA-BPD conference, the editors independently became concerned that the mental health field had failed to recognize the family's perspective on BPD. We both were aware that the families of patients with BPD were troubled by the same problems that traditionally vexed treaters: How much is the patient's accusatory anger due to me? If I do what's asked, am I collusive? If I refuse, am I being cruel? Why am I such an unsatisfactory caretaker? How can I be helpful? The resulting helplessness and inconsistencies, called "countertransference" problems when they occur in mental health professionals, are even more deeply demoralizing when they occur in families. Noting this, we both developed programs designed to help families and received funding from the National Institute of Mental Health (NIMH) to do this. Although the interventions we offered differed in some ways, participating families uniformly found great support from each other, felt empowered by knowledge about the disorder, and developed strong alliances with the treatment teams. These "veterans" became the members around whom local family advocacy organizations grew, one at the host hospital in the Boston area, McLean Hospital, and the other in Westchester County, New York.

The New England Personality Disorder Association (NEPDA) was founded in 1996. It subsequently became an essential component for the nationally based NEA-BPD, founded in August 2001. One of the initial statements made by the founders of NEA-BPD was, "We want to dispel some of the myths about BPD and bring hope to those affected by the disorder." This informal statement was formalized in the NEA-BPD mission statement: "To raise public awareness, provide education, promote research on borderline personality disorder, and enhance the quality of life of those affected by this serious mental illness." The goals and consequent activities of NEA-BPD stem from this mission: "To host annual conferences, provide family education programs, promote workshops, conduct family research, establish regional support centers for families, and publish educational materials and informational video-tapes."

Research on BPD is increasing in scope, and new treatments are being developed. To encourage young investigators, NEA-BPD, the National Alliance for Research on Schizophrenia and Depression (NARSAD), and the Borderline Personality Disorder Research Foundation (BPDRF) are co-sponsoring a Young Investigator Award (YIA). The award will be presented annually at the NEA-BPD conference and is supported by an R13 grant (R13 MH068456-01) from the National Institute of Mental Health. The YIA award is symbolic of NEA-BPD's determination to bring the work on BPD into the arena of public awareness.

There is still a long way to go. The work on BPD is 20 to 30 years behind that on other major psychiatric disorders such as depression and schizophrenia. Many who receive this diagnosis have to deal with family members and friends who, like them, have limited or no knowledge about the disorder. We hope that the balance of professional input and consumer and family experiences presented in this book will provide much-needed information and encouragement. Although we are particularly interested in families or patients themselves becoming educated, we are aware that much of what is in this book will be informative to mental health professionals as well. Our hope is that readers will learn more about BPD. We hope the information provided here will convey that BPD is a highly treatable disorder and that affected individuals can learn to lead full and rewarding lives.

One of the greatest tests in bringing this book to completion was to make it readable and meaningful for the widest possible audience. Recognizing our own limitations, we sought the talents of two experienced writer-educators, both non–mental health professionals, to help us meet the challenge. Working many months on the project, Penny Steiner-Grossman, Ed.D., M.P.H., designed and implemented a format that makes the book accessible to the lay person without compromising the quality and accuracy of the information needed by professionals. Patricia Woodward, M.A.T., who was involved from the book's inception, tirelessly guided the manuscript's development through its many iterations to ensure that deadlines were met and that American Psychiatric Association guidelines were satisfied. We extend our gratitude and appreciation to both of these devoted behind-the-scenes editors, whose skills made this book possible. We also acknowledge, with thanks, the superb contributions of Emily Neiditch, whose editing skills put the final touches on the manuscript.

All royalties from this publication will go to further the goals of the NEA-BPD and its work to help improve the lives of those affected by BPD—patients and family members alike.

John G. Gunderson, M.D.
Perry D. Hoffman, Ph.D.

A Word to the Lay Reader

This book was designed to provide useful information about borderline personality disorder for both professionals and lay readers. To make it more accessible to those without a background in psychology or psychiatry, we have set the more technical terms in each chapter in bold italic type and have defined those words at the end of the chapter in a section called "What Families Need to Know." This section also contains a summary of the key messages in the chapter, which we hope will clarify and reinforce the important points each author is making. We hope you will learn and understand more about borderline personality disorder from reading as much as possible of this book.

Part
I

Diagnosis, Treatment, and Prognosis

• 1 •

The Borderline Diagnosis

Concepts, Criteria, and Controversies

Andrew E. Skodol, M.D.

Borderline personality disorder (BPD) is a complex and serious mental disorder. It is estimated to occur in 1%–2% of the general population (Torgersen et al. 2001) and is the most common personality disorder for which people receive treatment. Ten percent of all psychiatric outpatients and 15%–20% of inpatients are estimated to have BPD (Widiger and Frances 1989). BPD is characterized by severe impairment in functioning (Skodol et al. 2002a), extensive use of psychiatric treatments (Bender et al. 2001), and a mortality rate by suicide of almost 10%—50 times higher than the rate in the general population (Work Group on Borderline Personality Disorder 2001). Nevertheless, effective treatments for BPD exist, and the *prognosis*—even over as short an interval as 1–2 years—may be better than expected (Gunderson et al. 2003; Shea et al. 2002).

From the perspectives of both the public and the mental health professional, BPD can also be a confusing and poorly understood disorder. In this chapter I describe the historical evolution of the concept of borderline personality to its current status as a personality disorder on *Axis II* of the assessment system that is outlined in the *Diagnostic and Statistical Manual of Mental Disorders,* 4th Edition, Text Revision (*DSM-IV-TR*) (American

Psychiatric Association 2000). I also review the current **diagnostic criteria** for BPD, as well as other manifestations that many believe are characteristic of the "borderline" patient. The chapter concludes with a discussion of several of the controversies that have surrounded the diagnosis of borderline personality over the years and that persist to this day.

● ● ●

Because of its associations with functional impairment, the need for hospitalization and for intensive outpatient treatment, self-destructive behaviors, and the potential for suicide, a diagnosis of BPD often provokes shock and despair in patients and families.

● ● ●

Borderline Concepts

The borderline concept dates back more than 60 years. Borderline patients were first described by Stern (1938) and later by Knight (1953). Kernberg (1967) referred to the intrapsychic features of these patients as "borderline personality organization," an intermediate level of internal personality organization more disturbed than that seen in a **neurotic** disorder but less disturbed than in a **psychotic** disorder. The notion that the disorder lay *between* the neurotic disorders and the psychotic disorders gave rise to the designation "borderline" in the first place. Borderline personality organization was characterized by an unstable sense of self (identity diffusion); use of primitive, immature **defense mechanisms** (categorizing others as "all good" or "all bad," denial, projection, acting out); and temporary lapses in the ability to distinguish the real from the imagined (defective reality testing). The Kernberg concept of borderline personality includes a number of other severe personality disorders as defined in DSM-IV-TR—for example, the narcissistic, antisocial, and schizoid types—in addition to BPD, a fact that has contributed to some of the confusion about the term.

The DSM definition of BPD arose from the work of Gunderson and Singer (1975), who identified from the literature characteristic unpleasant moods and emotions, impulsive actions, unstable interpersonal relations, psychotic-like thoughts, and social maladaptations. Several studies were then conducted to refine these descriptors so that they could be used to identify patients with BPD and also to discriminate such patients from those with other kinds of mental disorders (Gunderson and Kolb

1978; Spitzer et al. 1979). A final set of eight criteria was adopted for use in DSM-III (American Psychiatric Association 1980), the first official diagnostic manual to provide for the diagnosis of BPD (and all other mental disorders) by specified diagnostic criteria.

Diagnostic Criteria for BPD

Between the publication of DSM-III in 1980 and DSM-IV-TR in 2000, more than 300 studies were conducted on the criteria for arriving at a diagnosis of BPD. Some of these studies were done in an attempt to increase the precision with which BPD could be distinguished from other conditions, such as mood disorders or narcissistic personality disorders. The DSM-IV-TR criteria for BPD are listed in Table 1–1.

The essential features of BPD represent a pervasive pattern of marked *impulsivity* and instability in interpersonal relationships, self-image, and *affects* (moods and emotions). As with all personality disorders, these problems usually have their onset by late adolescence or early adulthood and are manifested in a variety of situations and life contexts.

● ● ●

BPD represents a pattern of impulsivity and instability in interpersonal relationships, self-image, and affects (moods and emotions).

● ● ●

Criterion 1 describes the frantic efforts people with BPD will make to avoid real or imagined abandonment by someone important to them. The perception of impending separation from an important other person has a destabilizing effect on the mood, sense of self, thought patterns, and behavior of the person with BPD. The person with BPD often misinterprets even the most realistic separations as rejections and indications that he or she is "bad."

Criterion 2 describes a pattern of intense and unstable relationships. People with BPD often become very involved with potential givers of care or love, even after a cursory meeting, and idealize the other person's virtues and capacities. If they are disappointed by that person, however, there can be a rapid shift to devaluing the other person, who now does not give or care nearly enough. Such dramatic shifts often occur in reaction to the perception of being rejected or abandoned.

Criterion 3 describes a disturbance in identity. The person with BPD can experience dramatic shifts in self-image characterized by shifting

Table 1–1. DSM-IV-TR diagnostic criteria for borderline personality disorder

A pervasive pattern of instability of interpersonal relationships, self-image, and affects, and marked impulsivity beginning by early adulthood and present in a variety of contexts, as indicated by five (or more) of the following:

(1) Frantic efforts to avoid real or imagined abandonment. Note: Do not include suicidal or self-mutilating behavior covered in Criterion 5.

(2) A pattern of unstable and intense interpersonal relationships characterized by alternating between extremes of idealization and devaluation

(3) Identity disturbance: markedly and persistently unstable self-image or sense of self

(4) Impulsivity in at least two areas that are potentially self-damaging (e.g., spending, sex, substance abuse, reckless driving, binge eating). Note: Do not include suicidal or self-mutilating behavior covered in Criterion 5.

(5) Recurrent suicidal behavior, gestures, or threats, or self-mutilating behavior

(6) Affective instability due to a marked reactivity of mood (e.g., intense episodic dysphoria, irritability, or anxiety usually lasting a few hours and only rarely more than a few days)

(7) Chronic feelings of emptiness

(8) Inappropriate, intense anger or difficulty controlling anger (e.g., frequent displays of temper, constant anger, recurrent physical fights)

(9) Transient, stress-related paranoid ideation or severe dissociative symptoms

Source. Reprinted from American Psychiatric Association: *Diagnostic and Statistical Manual of Mental Disorders*, 4th Edition, Text Revision. Washington, DC, American Psychiatric Association, 2000. Copyright 2000, American Psychiatric Association. Used with permission.

goals, values, aspirations, friends, sexual identity, etc. Patients with BPD often feel bad or evil and sometimes as if they do not exist at all, particularly in situations in which they perceive inadequate nurturing and support from others.

Criterion 4 describes self-damaging impulsivity. Individuals with BPD frequently abuse substances, engage in unsafe sex, binge eat, gamble, overspend money, or drive recklessly. Patients with BPD also make impulsive suicide threats or gestures and may self-mutilate by cutting themselves with a razor blade or burning themselves with cigarettes. These behaviors are also frequently precipitated by separation, rejection, or the expectation that the individuals will assume greater responsibility for themselves than they are accustomed to. These behaviors are described by criterion 5.

People with BPD experience marked shifts in their moods and other emotions. They may experience depression, irritability, anxiety, anger, panic, or despair—often lasting only a few hours—usually in reaction to interpersonal stresses. This affective instability is described by criterion 6. Criterion 7 describes the chronic feelings of emptiness and boredom often experienced by patients with BPD. Criterion 8 describes the intense and inappropriate anger they often feel and express toward others whom they perceive as being neglectful, withholding, uncaring, and abandoning. Under extreme stress, a person with BPD may become temporarily paranoid and suspicious or may *dissociate,* so that he or she feels detached from his or her own thinking or body. The stressor again is commonly perceived abandonment. These reactions are described by criterion 9.

Given that any five of these nine diagnostic criteria can substantiate a diagnosis of BPD, it is readily apparent that there are many combinations of symptoms (126 to be exact) that can characterize individuals with BPD. This heterogeneity has led to a search for core underlying dimensions of psychopathology that all patients with BPD share. The most commonly suggested core structure consists of three basic disturbances: disturbed interpersonal relatedness, affective or emotional *dysregulation,* and behavioral dyscontrol or impulsivity (Sanislow et al. 2002). The search is on to try to discover the genetic, neurobiological, and environmental bases for these core disturbances (Skodol et al. 2002b, 2002c).

Several other traits not exactly represented by the diagnostic criteria are thought by some experts to also be characteristic of BPD. One is a tendency to regress (i.e., to adopt childish behaviors and expectations) when placed in situations where what is expected of them is not clearly delineated. The primitive defenses described in Kernberg's borderline personality organization concept are only indirectly represented by the DSM-IV-TR criteria of interpersonal problems, impulsiveness, and stress-related paranoia and dissociation. Because of their feelings of extremely insecure attachment, patients with BPD often cling not only to people in real life, but also to objects that they associate with people, such as a stuffed animal (so-called transitional objects). Future versions of the DSM may well include additional or alternative criteria to describe the essence of these characteristic borderline traits.

● ● ●

When BPD occurs with other disorders, such as anxiety or mood disorders, this often complicates the treatment of these conditions and leads to a poorer outcome.

● ● ●

Borderline personality disorder can coexist with other mental disorders, including other personality disorders. When BPD occurs with other disorders, such as anxiety or **mood disorders,** this often complicates the treatment of these conditions and leads to a poorer outcome. In addition, although BPD shares some features with other personality disorders, it can be distinguished from those disorders. For example, patients with histrionic personality disorder may be attention seeking and manipulative and may have shifting emotions, but they do not show the intense anger, have feelings of emptiness, or exhibit the destructive impulsivity of patients with BPD. Those with schizotypal personality disorder are often paranoid or experience perceptual distortions, but these symptoms are not as transitory as those experienced by patients with BPD. People with paranoid or narcissistic personality disorders may react with intense anger when they feel slighted, but they do not exhibit the self-destructive impulsivity or have the abandonment fears of the person with BPD. Patients with antisocial personality disorder manipulate others, but it is usually for material gain, rather than to be taken care of as is the case with BPD. Individuals with dependent personality disorder may fear separation from a close other, but will not react with rage, feelings of emptiness, and manipulative suicide attempts like the person with BPD.

Controversies About the Borderline Diagnosis

In this section I discuss five controversial issues concerning the borderline diagnosis: 1) its relationship with other disorders, 2) its reliability, 3) its gender distribution, 4) its **etiology,** and 5) its prognosis.

On the Border With What?

The term *borderline* originated from the psychoanalytic notion of a level of personality organization that was in between, or on the border of, the psychotic and the neurotic disorders. Although BPD has become of interest to mainstream psychiatry and psychology and is no longer solely a psychoanalytic **construct,** the name *borderline* has persisted; the search continues for other mental disorders that lie along the border with BPD.

An early hypothesis was that BPD represented patients with borderline schizophrenia. The Danish Adoption Study of Schizophrenia (Kety et al. 1968) identified a **cohort** of patients with a nonpsychotic form of schizophrenia who had a genetic relationship to schizophrenic parents. Features describing these patients were included in Spitzer and colleagues' (1979) **empirical** attempt to identify diagnostic criteria for BPD.

These traits of deficits in interpersonal relatedness and peculiarities of *ideation,* appearance, and behavior eventually came to describe the characteristics of schizotypal personality disorder, whereas BPD itself continues to be associated more with the borderline concept that grew from the psychoanalytic literature.

The next wave of research raised the issue of whether BPD was an atypical form of mood disorder. Because of the rapidly shifting mood states that characterize individuals with BPD, the latest version of this controversy is that BPD represents a treatment-**refractory,** rapid-cycling form of atypical bipolar II disorder (with only **hypomanic** or low-level mania experienced, not full-blown mania). Although this theory has led to the frequent prescription of mood-stabilizing medications, which can be helpful for the affective instability in some cases, the bulk of the evidence fails to support the equivalence of BPD and any mood disorder (Gunderson and Phillips 1991). Although it is certain that mood disturbance and diagnosable mood disorder may coexist with BPD, mood disorder alone cannot account for the fears of abandonment, the particular types of interpersonal relatedness, and the impulsivity of BPD patients.

Most recently, the interest in childhood abuse as an etiological factor in BPD and the prevalence of posttraumatic stress disorder (**PTSD**) as a **comorbid** (or co-occurring) condition have led to studies investigating whether BPD was a variant of PTSD. Here too, research has shown that PTSD and BPD have certain features in common but that the psychopathology and functioning of BPD cannot be reduced to a variant of PTSD (Gunderson and Sabo 1993; Zlotnick et al. 2003).

● ● ●

*The term **borderline** has also been used pejoratively to describe patients who "misbehave" or are difficult to treat because of their extremes of behavior and the fact that therapists often become entwined in their interpersonal problems.*

● ● ●

A corollary to the search for a border disorder for BPD has been the search for a new name. If it is true that BPD is not really a variant of or on the border with any other major mental disorder but is a major disorder in its own right, perhaps the borderline concept has outlived its usefulness and ought to be replaced with a more descriptively accurate and potentially more useful term. The term *borderline* has also been used pejoratively to describe patients who "misbehave" or are difficult to treat because of their extremes of behavior and the fact that therapists often become entwined in their interpersonal problems. The most commonly suggested alternative names are *emotional dysregulation disorder* and *emotional regulation disorder,* which have been suggested by those who consider affective instability to be the core disturbance of BPD; the name *emotional/impulse (dys)regulation disorder* has been suggested by those who argue that at least two core disturbances exist: affective instability *and* impulse control. Because the fundamental basis of the disorder is not understood, there do not appear to be clear scientific grounds to resolve the controversy over a name change. Therefore, because the diagnosis of BPD has acquired widespread clinical usage and is recognized by clinicians who deal with patients with personality disorder as a clinically useful construct, its name will probably remain unchanged for the immediate future.

Can BPD Be Diagnosed Reliably?

Reliability refers to the reproducibility of a measurement or assessment from one assessor or occasion to another. It has often been claimed that two clinicians cannot agree on whether a patient has BPD or not (i.e., that it cannot be diagnosed reliably). This impression may result from the different meanings of the term *borderline,* because the concept has evolved from its psychoanalytic origins to its DSM-IV-TR definition. The combination of a definition by specific diagnostic criteria, making explicit the signs and symptoms of the disorder, with the standardized interview schedules developed to collect relevant symptom information should ensure the reliability of the BPD diagnosis.

The Collaborative Longitudinal Personality Disorders Study (CLPS), funded by the National Institute of Mental Health, used a standardized interview to assess all DSM-IV (American Psychiatric Association 1994) personality disorders (Zanarini et al. 2000). In this study and in another using an interview designed exclusively to assess BPD symptoms (Zanarini et al. 2002), the reliability of the BPD diagnosis and most of its individual symptoms was very good to excellent. The high levels of reliability found in both of these studies are consistent with the results of other studies using standardized interviews and diagnosis by criteria; they are as high as or higher than those for many other mental disorders for which the reliability of diagnosis is seldom questioned. Of course, standardized interviews and specified criteria are not synonymous with excellent clinical judgment, and unless clinicians are well trained in the diagnosis of BPD, reliability of the diagnosis will be less than optimal.

Is BPD a Gender-Biased Diagnosis?

According to DSM-IV-TR, BPD is "diagnosed predominantly (about 75%) in females" (American Psychiatric Association 2000, p. 708). A female-to-male gender ratio of 3:1 is quite striking for a mental disorder and suggests the possibility of sampling or diagnostic bias or of biological or sociocultural differences between women and men that lead to the development of BPD.

A sampling bias can occur if the proportion of women with BPD is no greater than the proportion of women versus men seen in a clinical setting. If women were three times more likely to seek help for psychological problems, then it would be no surprise that the disorders found would appear on average to be three times more common in women. Most studies in clinics that have used standardized interview assessments have found no greater proportion of women with BPD than of all women treated in the setting, suggesting that a sampling bias may account for at least some of the higher observed prevalence of BPD in women. There are as yet too few studies of BPD in the general population to know what the real gender ratio may be.

Diagnostic biases may exist if the construct of BPD or its criteria reflect a sexist characterization of female behavior as pathological, or if women exhibiting the same traits or behaviors as men would be more likely to be labeled as abnormal. Another diagnostic bias would exist if errors in making the diagnosis of BPD were more common for female patients than for male patients. A number of studies have shown that BPD criteria, except anger, may be considered slightly more characteristic of women than of men (Sprock et al. 1990) and more pathological in women (Sprock 1996). A study by Johnson et al. (2003) showed that women and men with BPD are more similar than different. Women may demonstrate their impulsivity differently than men do—for example, by engaging in binge eating rather than substance abuse. Also, female patients receive unwarranted diagnoses of BPD more often than do male patients, but, surprisingly perhaps to the gender-bias theorists, misdiagnosis occurs more often when the clinician is also a woman. Although there is modest support for diagnostic biases of various kinds, none of these are strong enough to account for the wide difference in prevalence reported. If the true prevalence rate of BPD in women is higher than that in men, it would have to be the result of biological or sociocultural factors. Among the possible risk factors for BPD (Table 1–2), some have been found to be more common in women. For example, the personality trait of neuroticism (emotionality, impulsivity, vulnerability to stress), which is thought to underlie BPD and is under genetic influence, occurs more frequently in women. Childhood sexual abuse, which has been implicated in the genesis of BPD, is 10 times more common in women than in men. Different rearing practices lead boys to develop more externalizing, action-oriented ways of dealing with problems and stress, whereas girls are often reared to be more internalizing and emotional. Future studies are needed to shed light on gender differences in biological and social processes that may foster the development of BPD.

Is Nature or Nurture More Important in the Etiology of BPD?

As indicated in Table 1–2, because risk factors are derived from both biological and sociocultural realms, there are diverse theories about the etiology of BPD. Some scientists believe that the essential features of BPD are best explained on the basis of genetic inheritance of neurobiological abnormalities, whereas others focus on a history of adverse experiences.

BPD itself has recently been shown to be *heritable.* A twin study in Norway (Torgersen et al. 2000) found a *concordance* for definite BPD of 35% in monozygotic (identical) twin pairs compared with 7% in dizygotic (fraternal) pairs. Subthreshold BPD was concordant in 38% of monozygotic and 11% of dizygotic pairs. A genetic model yielded a heritability effect of 0.69 (1.0 would indicate complete heritability), suggesting there is a strong genetic component in the development of BPD.

Table 1–2.   Potential risk factors for borderline personality disorder

Genes
Childhood temperament or predispositions
Autonomic nervous system arousal and reactivity
Neurotransmitter responsivity
Brain structure and functioning
Perinatal factors
Hormones
Environmental toxins
Cognitive and other neuropsychological factors
Prior childhood or adolescent psychopathology
Personality structure or traits
Faulty or inadequate parenting approaches
Child abuse or neglect
Peer influences
Socioeconomic status
Family and community disintegration

As mentioned in the preceding section, the personality trait of neuroticism, which includes emotionality and impulsivity, has been shown to be heritable. Other twin studies have demonstrated substantial heritability for other traits of BPD such as anxiety, affective **lability,** cognitive dysregulation, identity problems, and insecure attachment (Jang et al. 1996; Livesley et al. 1993). These traits can be included in a large category called emotional dysregulation, which represents many, but not all, traits of BPD. Biological studies have shown that affective instability is associated with increased responsivity of brain cholinergic and adrenergic systems and that impulsivity is associated with decreased activity of the neurotransmitter **serotonin** in the brain. These abnormalities in brain systems may underlie the personality traits that have been shown to be heritable.

● ● ●

A sensible hypothesis provides for a model in which genetic predispositions interact with environmental stressors to produce the disorder.

● ● ●

Adverse experiences during childhood, such as loss of a parent before age 16 or poor or negligent parenting, have also been implicated in the development of personality disorders, including BPD. The most frequent finding for parenting in individuals with personality disorder has been a serious problem in bonding with parents because of both a lack of affection (neglect) and a lack of autonomy (overcontrol) (Paris et al. 1994a, 1994b). These findings are not specific for BPD, however. Those with BPD also report low family cohesion (Feldman et al. 1995; Ogata et al. 1990a). Retrospective reports of childhood sexual and/or physical abuse are also particularly common among patients with BPD (Herman et al. 1989; Links et al 1988; Ogata et al. 1990b; Paris et al. 1994a, 1994b). But even child trauma is not very specific for BPD. Furthermore, community studies of child abuse in the general population indicate that 80% of adults with abuse histories do not develop any kind of psychopathology.

It is evident that a simple explanation for the causes of BPD will not be viable. A more sensible hypothesis provides for a model in which certain genetic predispositions (personality traits, biological vulnerabilities) interact with certain environmental stressors (psychosocial risk factors) to produce the disorder. This *diathesis-stress model* was first suggested for BPD by Stone (1980) and has been developed further by Paris (1999) and others. An unusual intensity of certain vulnerability traits would lower the threshold for the magnitude of the stressors that could result in BPD. In addition, personality disorders most likely involve gene–environment interactions, in which some of the underlying traits increase both exposure and susceptibility to environmental stressors. The temperamental precursors of both impulsivity and affective instability are likely to increase the chances that children will be mistreated and that mistreatment will cause overt problems with impulse control and mood disturbance.

Is the Prognosis for BPD Hopeless?

Because of its associations with impairment in functioning, the need for hospitalization and intensive outpatient treatment, self-destructive behavior, and the potential for suicide, a diagnosis of BPD often provokes shock and despair in patients and families. However, follow-up studies of individuals who receive a diagnosis of BPD suggest that the prognosis is not as grave as is often presumed. A review of 13 studies of the stability of a BPD diagnosis made according to specified criteria and with the assistance of a standardized interview (Skodol et al. 2002b) revealed that only about half of the subjects retained the diagnosis. The lowest stability was found among patients who were diagnosed in adolescence, a time when personality is often considered to be in flux. In general, the longer the follow-up period, the greater the chance for improvement (McDavid and Pilkonis 1996; Perry 1993). In the prospective follow-along CLPS study, 10% of those diagnosed with BPD showed dramatic improvement within the first 6 months of follow-up, and resolution of a co-occurring mental disorder or a psychosocial or interpersonal crisis played a major role in the improvement (Gunderson et al. 2003). Only 41% of BPD patients met full criteria every month for the first year (Shea et al. 2002). Poor prognostic factors include a history of childhood sexual abuse and incest; early age at first psychiatric contact; impulsivity, aggression, and substance abuse; and greater severity and chronicity of symptoms (Skodol et al. 2002b). Nonetheless, the prognosis of BPD is clearly not as poor as has generally been believed.

Conclusion

The borderline diagnosis has a long history in psychiatry. Over the past quarter-century, it has come to identify a complex and serious mental disorder. The identification of BPD by specified diagnostic criteria has allowed the diagnosis to be made reliably and has opened doors to serious research into its significance, its causes, and its treatment. Although BPD is associated with significant functional impairment, extensive use of psychiatric treatments, and an increased risk of suicide, its prognosis—at least in some cases—may be better than has generally been believed.

What Families Need to Know

Key Messages in This Chapter

- Borderline personality disorder (BPD) is a serious and complex disorder affecting an estimated 1%–2% of the general population.
- The name *borderline* refers to the original notion that the disorder lies in between or on the border with the psychotic and neurotic mental disorders.
- The core symptoms common to most people with BPD are disturbed, unstable relationships with other people; emotional dysregulation (the inability to control mood or feelings); and impulsive behavior.
- Although BPD has some features in common with other personality disorders and with mood disorders (such as anxiety and depression), it is distinct from them.
- Women receive a diagnosis of BPD more frequently than men do, and this may be the result of biological and sociocultural factors. A partial explanation of this difference may be that women seek help more often than men for psychological problems.
- Although early reports suggested that those with BPD had a history of physical or sexual abuse, large-scale studies of child abuse in the general population show that 80% of adults with abuse histories do not develop any psychological problems.
- The current hypothesis (theory) suggests that individuals may be genetically prone to developing BPD and that certain stressful events may trigger the onset of BPD.

Key Words in This Chapter

affective   pertaining to one's emotional state.

Axis II   a classification in DSM-IV-TR for personality disorders, for example, borderline personality disorder.

cohort   a group of similar individuals studied over time.

comorbid   occurring together with another disease or condition.

concordance   having the same diagnosis, as in the study of a condition occurring in twins, suggesting that the condition may be inherited.

construct an idea or concept made up of separate parts.

defense mechanisms unconscious reactions (such as denial) used to resolve or conceal conflicts or anxieties.

diagnostic criteria a list of clinical features that must be present for the diagnosis of a mental disorder to be made.

diathesis-stress model a model in which genetic predispositions interact with environmental stressors to produce the disorder.

dissociation feelings of detachment from one's own body or thinking.

DSM-IV-TR *Diagnostic and Statistical Manual of Mental Disorders,* 4th Edition, Text Revision, a system of classification of psychiatric diagnoses published in 2000.

dysregulation the inability to regulate or control mood.

empirical based on evidence, data, or experience.

etiology cause or presumed cause.

heritable capable of being inherited.

hypomanic having an abnormally elevated mood and level of activity (restlessness) leading to some interference with daily living.

ideation the process of thinking or forming ideas.

impulsivity inability to resist performing some action.

lability rapid fluctuation; instability, changeability.

mood disorders a group of disorders (including depression and bipolar disorder) in which a disturbance of mood is accompanied by impaired cognitive function and physical signs, such as disturbed sleep, or changes in appetite and level of energy.

neurosis a chronic or recurrent nonpsychotic disorder characterized mainly by anxiety.

prognosis prediction about the future course of a condition, including the chance for recovery or relapse.

psychosis a loss of reality testing and impairment of mental, social, and personal functioning.

PTSD posttraumatic stress disorder.

refractory resistant to treatment.

serotonin a neurotransmitter or brain chemical that can regulate affective symptoms (mood) and impulsive behavior.

References

American Psychiatric Association: Diagnostic and Statistical Manual of Mental Disorders, 3rd Edition. Washington, DC, American Psychiatric Association, 1980

American Psychiatric Association: Diagnostic and Statistical Manual of Mental Disorders, 4th Edition. Washington, DC, American Psychiatric Association, 1994

American Psychiatric Association: Diagnostic and Statistical Manual of Mental Disorders, 4th Edition, Text Revision. Washington, DC, American Psychiatric Association, 2000

Bender DS, Dolan RT, Skodol AE, et al: Treatment utilization by patients with personality disorders. Am J Psychiatry 158:295–302, 2001

Feldman RB, Zelkowitz P, Weiss M, et al: A comparison of the families of borderline personality disorder mothers and the families of other personality disorder mothers. Compr Psychiatry 36:157–163, 1995

Gunderson JG, Kolb JE: Discriminating features of borderline patients. Am J Psychiatry 135:792–796, 1978

Gunderson JG, Phillips KA: A current view of the interface between borderline personality disorder and depression. Am J Psychiatry 148:967–975, 1991

Gunderson JG, Sabo AN: The phenomenological and conceptual interface between borderline personality disorder and PTSD. Am J Psychiatry 150:19–27, 1993

Gunderson JG, Singer MT: Defining borderline patients: an overview. Am J Psychiatry 132:1–10, 1975

Gunderson JG, Bender D, Sanislow C, et al: Plausibility and possible determinants of sudden "remissions" in borderline patients. Psychiatry 66:111–119, 2003

Herman JL, Perry JC, van der Kolk BA: Childhood trauma in borderline personality disorder. Am J Psychiatry 146:490–495, 1989

Jang KL, Livesley WJ, Vernon PA, et al: Heritability of personality disorder traits: a twin study. Acta Psychiatr Scand 94:438–444, 1996

Johnson DM, Shea MT, Yen S, et al: Gender differences in borderline personality disorder: findings from the Collaborative Longitudinal Personality Disorders Study. Compr Psychiatry 44:284–292, 2003

Kernberg OF: Borderline personality organization. J Am Psychoanal Assoc 15:641–685, 1967

Kety SS, Rosenthal D, Wender PH, et al: The types and prevalences of mental illness in the biological and adoptive families of adopted schizophrenics, in The Transmission of Schizophrenia. Edited by Rosenthal D, Kety SS. London, Pergamon, 1968, pp 345–362

Knight R: Borderline states. Bull Menninger Clin 17:1–12, 1953

Links PS, Steiner M, Offord DR: Characteristics of borderline personality disorder: a Canadian study. Can J Psychiatry 33:336–340, 1988

Livesley WJ, Jang KL, Jackson DN, et al: Genetic and environmental contributions to dimensions of personality disorder. Am J Psychiatry 150:1826–1831, 1993

McDavid JD, Pilkonis PA: The stability of personality disorder diagnosis. J Personal Disord 10:1–15, 1996

Ogata SN, Silk KR, Goodrich S: The childhood experience of the borderline patient, in Family Environment and Borderline Personality Disorder. Edited by Links PS. Washington, DC, American Psychiatric Press, 1990a, pp 87–103

Ogata SN, Silk KR, Goodrich S: Childhood sexual and physical abuse in adult patients with borderline personality disorder. Am J Psychiatry 147:1008–1013, 1990b

Paris J: Nature and Nurture in Psychiatry: A Predisposition-Stress Model of Mental Disorders. Washington, DC, American Psychiatric Press, 1999

Paris J, Zweig-Frank H, Guzder J: Psychological risk factors for borderline personality disorder in female patients. Compr Psychiatry 35:301–305, 1994a

Paris J, Zweig-Frank H, Guzder J: Risk factors for borderline personality in male outpatients. J Nerv Ment Dis 182:375–380, 1994b

Perry JC: Longitudinal studies of personality disorders. J Personal Disord 7:63–85, 1993

Sanislow CA, Grilo CM, Morey LC, et al: Confirmatory factor analysis of DSM-IV criteria for borderline personality disorder: findings from the Collaborative Longitudinal Personality Disorders Study. Am J Psychiatry 159:284–290, 2002

Shea MT, Stout R, Gunderson J, et al: Short-term diagnostic stability of schizotypal, borderline, avoidant, and obsessive-compulsive personality disorders. Am J Psychiatry 159:2036–2041, 2002

Skodol AE, Gunderson JG, McGlashan TH, et al: Functional impairment in patients with schizotypal, borderline, avoidant, or obsessive-compulsive personality disorder. Am J Psychiatry 159:276–283, 2002a

Skodol AE, Gunderson JG, Pfohl B, et al: The borderline diagnosis I: psychopathology, comorbidity, and personality structure. Biol Psychiatry 51:936–950, 2002b

Skodol AE, Siever LJ, Livesley WJ, et al: The borderline diagnosis II: biology, genetics, and clinical course. Biol Psychiatry 51:951–963, 2002c

Spitzer RL, Endicott J, Gibbon M: Crossing the border into borderline personality and borderline schizophrenia: the development of criteria. Arch Gen Psychiatry 36:17–24, 1979

Sprock J: Abnormality ratings of the DSM-III-R personality disorder criteria for males vs. females. J Nerv Ment Dis 184:314–316, 1996

Sprock J, Blashfield RK, Smith B: Gender weighting of DSM-III-R personality disorder criteria. Am J Psychiatry 147:586–590, 1990

Stern A: Psychoanalytic investigation and therapy in the borderline group of neuroses. Psychoanal Q 7:467–489, 1938

Stone MH: The Borderline Syndromes. New York, McGraw-Hill, 1980

Torgersen S, Lygren S, Øien PA, et al: A twin study of personality disorders. Compr Psychiatry 41:416–425, 2000

Torgersen S, Kringlen E, Cramer V: The prevalence of personality disorders in a community sample. Arch Gen Psychiatry 58:590–596, 2001

Widiger TA, Frances AJ: Epidemiology, diagnosis, and comorbidity of borderline personality disorder, in American Psychiatric Press Review of Psychiatry, Vol 8. Edited by Tasman A, Hales RE, Frances AJ. Washington, DC, American Psychiatric Press, 1989, pp 8–24

Work Group on Borderline Personality Disorder: Practice guideline for the treatment of patients with borderline personality disorder. Am J Psychiatry 158 (suppl):1–52, 2001

Zanarini MC, Skodol AE, Bender DS, et al: The Collaborative Longitudinal Personality Disorders Study: reliability of Axis I and Axis II diagnoses. J Personal Disord 14:291–299, 2000

Zanarini MC, Frankenburg FR, Vujanovic AA: Inter-rater and test-retest reliability of the Revised Diagnostic Interview for Borderlines. J Personal Disord 16:270–276, 2002

Zlotnick C, Johnson DM, Yen S, et al: Clinical features and impairment in women with borderline personality disorder (BPD) with posttraumatic stress disorder (PTSD), BPD without PTSD, and other personality disorders with PTSD. J Nerv Ment Dis 191:706–713, 2003

• 2 •

Psychotherapies for Borderline Personality Disorder

Donna S. Bender, Ph.D.
John M. Oldham, M.D.

In 2001, after considerable deliberation and extensive involvement by a number of experts in the field, the American Psychiatric Association adopted its "Practice Guideline for the Treatment of Patients With Borderline Personality Disorder" (American Psychiatric Association 2001). In the guideline, psychotherapy is recommended as the core treatment for borderline personality disorder (BPD): "Most patients with borderline personality disorder will need extended psychotherapy in order to attain and maintain lasting improvement in their personality, interpersonal problems, and overall functioning" (p. 4). This having been established, one must consider that there are a number of possible psychotherapy options. The purpose of this chapter is to review outpatient psychotherapy treatments for BPD.

Acknowledgments: Nancee Blum (Systems Training for Emotional Predictability and Problem Solving), Department of Psychiatry, University of Iowa; Monica Carsky (Psychoanalytically Informed Supportive Psychotherapy) and Frank Yeomans (Transference-Focused Psychotherapy), New York Presbyterian Hospital Personality Disorders Institute.

History of Treatment

Borderline personality was not defined as a disorder per se until the 1970s, although the *constellation* of symptoms, or syndrome, had been described as a challenge to the mental health field for many decades before that. As Knight (1953/1989) noted, "The term 'borderline state' has achieved almost no official status in the psychiatric *nomenclature*, and conveys no diagnostic illumination of a case other than the implication that the person is quite sick but not frankly psychotic" (p. 96). Originally, the transient *psychotic* episodes, rapidly shifting mental states, and lack of response to treatment led some to associate these types of patients with the schizophrenia spectrum disorders. However, the same patients could at times appear like higher-functioning *neurotic* patients. Thus there was considerable debate about the nature of this type of disturbance, which was sometimes seen as being on the border between schizophrenia and neurosis—hence the term *borderline* (M. H. Stone 1977). As a result, there were a number of different responses by treaters.

● ● ●

In retrospect, some of Freud's patients probably would be considered borderline by today's definitions, and there have always been creative and skilled analysts and therapists who have worked successfully with these types of problems.

● ● ●

In retrospect, some of Freud's patients probably would be considered borderline by today's definitions, and there have always been creative and skilled analysts and therapists who have worked successfully with these types of problems. However, the classical technique associated with American psychoanalysis in the 1950s and 1960s proved ineffective—and sometimes detrimental—in the treatment of many patients with borderline issues. With interpretation as the cornerstone intervention (one that is often not very well tolerated by these individuals in the first phase of analysis), prolonged silences by the analyst were experienced by the patient as abandonment. There was also little room for tumultuous acting out in the narrow verbal confines of the "talking cure" being practiced at that time. Therefore, for quite a while, medical psychoanalysis viewed patients with BPD as being too disturbed to be treated in analysis.

At the same time, a subgroup of analysts had begun to directly consider the applicability of psychoanalysis to more disturbed patients. The so-called widening scope of psychoanalysis (L. Stone 1954) saw the introduction of theoretical and technical modifications and innovations that now make psychoanalysis and psychodynamic psychotherapy the treatment of choice for many individuals with BPD. During the 1970s, borderline issues increasingly became part of mainstream psychology and psychiatry considerations, particularly as a result of the efforts of Otto Kernberg (e.g., Kernberg 1967, 1975, 1976) to further both clinical and empirical discourse centered on these issues. With this rise in attention to borderline conditions, a number of specialized treatments were also developed. Along with specific *psychodynamic psychotherapies, cognitive-behavioral therapies* that were previously used for problems such as depression and anxiety have now been adapted to personality disorders as well.

General Considerations for Therapy

Although in subsequent sections of this chapter we describe several broad traditions of treatment and specific approaches within each, we begin by discussing several issues to be considered regardless of the treatment chosen. Individuals with BPD are likely to present for treatment with impaired coping strategies; troubled relationships; and related difficulties such as anxiety, substance abuse, and depression. In addition, there are different types of individuals for whom the term *borderline* may be applicable, as well as shifts in the prominence of particular issues as treatment progresses. As a result, different psychotherapeutic approaches may be desirable for different patients, or the same patient may use different treatments over time.

The first priority, transcending treatment approach, is to ensure that the patient is not in danger of hurting him- or herself or others. Gunderson (2001) outlined recommendations for assessing the level of care appropriate for an individual patient dealing with specific types of issues. Suicidal thoughts and self-mutilation behavior must be monitored as carefully as possible, and in cases of potential serious harm, a referral to an inpatient setting may be necessary. In addition, the therapist also must consistently attend to symptoms and behaviors that may threaten the integrity and continuity of the treatment itself. It may be appropriate to use *adjunctive* therapies such as psychiatric medications for anxiety, depression, psychotic episodes, and mood instability, as well as specific substance abuse programs if the substance use is substantially interfering with the psychotherapeutic work (American Psychiatric Association 2001).

• • •

*Although establishing an alliance is important
in all types of treatments for patients with all
types of problems, it is of fundamental importance in working with individuals with BPD.*

• • •

After those first-line considerations have been addressed, the second
fundamental long-term goal is to assist individuals with BPD in developing more flexible thought and behavior patterns to replace unconstruc-
tive and harmful ways of being. To accomplish these broad goals, the
clinician must be able to engage the patient in a constructive therapeutic
endeavor. This is true whether the therapist works within a psychoana-
lytic/psychodynamic model or practices cognitive-behavioral treatment.

Although establishing an **alliance** is important in all types of treatments for patients with all types of presenting problems, it is of fundamental importance in working with individuals with BPD issues. As Bach
(1998) noted, for a complex set of reasons many of these patients "have
generally lost their faith not only in their caregivers, spouses, and other
objects (people), but also in the world itself as a place of expectable and
manageable contingencies" (p. 185). Therefore, forming an alliance is
often difficult, because troubled and greatly fluctuating interpersonal attitudes and behaviors associated with BPD may also infuse the patient's
engagement with the therapist, possibly thwarting the potential helpful-
ness of the treater. Therefore, when one is looking for a clinician who
treats BPD, it is important to assess to the extent possible the goodness
of fit between the patient and therapist. That is, as difficult as it may be
to contemplate entering into a treatment relationship—and for some patients with BPD it may be acutely so—there must be some sense on the
patient's part that he or she can establish a working relationship with the
treater. This is also the case because any potentially effective psychotherapy is likely to have a fairly long duration, so one would hope to be able
to feel some comfort in making a commitment.

It is recommended that the patient schedule multiple consultation
sessions with the prospective therapist, attending to several important issues during these meetings: level of comfort in speaking with the therapist, some understanding and acceptance of the therapist's approach,
and the sense that the therapist is competent in treating BPD issues. Although it is often helpful to obtain referrals from a respected source, one
should not make a commitment to treatment solely on that basis. Even
though the therapist may be well known or the referring party is of es-

teemed stature, these factors do not guarantee that the approach or the therapist's personal style will suit a particular individual.

It should also be noted that some of the therapies include participation in group skills training, which can be a very helpful additional component of treatment. However, as with choosing an individual therapist, it is important to understand what is entailed in this type of program. Certain individuals may have a very difficult time engaging in a group format or may have expectations that cannot be met by the group. One should consider these factors before committing to such a treatment.

Outpatient Psychotherapies

Establishing an ongoing and productive working relationship with a therapist is a fundamental goal in any treatment, but it is of particular importance for individuals with BPD because it is often very difficult to facilitate with these patients. Consequently, therapists practicing a wide variety of therapy disciplines have recognized the importance of employing a supportive stance with their borderline patients. Winston and colleagues (2001) advocated the notion that "supportive therapy can be considered a 'shell' that fits over most theoretical orientations" (p. 346). That is, whether the core orientation of the treatment is from a cognitive-behavioral or a psychodynamic tradition (both of which are described in this chapter), a supportive demeanor is necessary to engage and keep the patient in treatment. Although it is important in establishing the alliance, this approach also allows the therapist to model an alternative way of interacting through such interventions as empathic responses and validation of feelings. The therapy relationship is used to teach the patient about his or her difficulties with other people, to enhance the patient's self-esteem, and to assist in managing anxiety. A variety of psychotherapeutic approaches have incorporated supportive elements in treating patients with BPD, and many therapists now employ supportive psychotherapy as a distinct approach in and of itself.

Psychodynamic Psychotherapies and Psychoanalysis: General Description

The psychodynamic/psychoanalytic approach generally focuses on enduring patterns of thoughts, emotions, and behaviors that may or may not be in conscious awareness. Because the patient's difficulties frequently become manifest in the treatment room, making them directly available for consideration, the relationship between patient and therapist is used as a primary vehicle for change. This is the case not only in terms of working with the *transference* (old wishes, expectations, and conflicts that shape current relationships) but also in using the relationship itself as a positive model for identification and emulation. It is usually recommended that individuals with BPD attend therapy more than once a week. Psychodynamic psychotherapy is informed by psychoanalytic theory. Psychoanalysis is considered to be a more intensive form of treatment compared with psychotherapy because it most often entails four or more sessions a week. Lying on the couch is also usually part of the process of psychoanalysis, and there is some controversy about using this method in the treatment of borderline patients. This group of patients is very heterogeneous: some are able to use the couch to good effect; others are able to do it after a first phase of treatment conducted sitting up; and still others may have great difficulty working in treatment in this manner.

How the therapist interacts with the patient and chooses the kinds of interventions depends on the particular types of issues that are most salient for the individual patient. The approach may vary according to the patient's needs in any given session or during different phases of the treatment. Gabbard (2000) emphasized the importance of understanding that there is usually a mixture of expressive and supportive elements in every analysis or psychodynamic psychotherapy. That is, the expressive, insight-oriented mode of assisting patients in uncovering unconscious conflicts, thoughts, or emotions through interpretation may be appropriate at times, whereas a more supportive approach of bolstering the patient's coping abilities is preferable in other circumstances. Some individuals with BPD may not be able to tolerate a discussion of unconscious motivations in the earlier phase of treatment because this may be experienced as too intrusive or as impinging on acute vulnerabilities. Therefore, supportive, empathic communications may be more effective interventions in building an alliance by helping the patient feel heard and understood. This phase of the treatment could go on for quite some time before the patient is capable of participating in a more expressive mode of treatment. During the course of treatment, there may be periods when the patient once again needs predominantly supportive interventions. A skilled therapist will be flexible, moving back and forth along the expressive-supportive continuum as needed by the individual patient.

Use of Theoretical Models in Treating BPD

Therapeutic work is also guided by the clinician's use of various theoretical models about the etiology of character pathology. Although psychoanalytic theories about the nature of psychopathology and its treatment abound, we mention only some of the main approaches here. Many who work with BPD patients use an object relations perspective that views the individual's earliest experiences and relationships as focal points for understanding the salient features of how he or she relates to others as an adult (Pine 1990). (For historical reasons in the psychoanalytic literature, the term *object* refers to the person.) Central to this way of thinking is that all people construct mental representations of self-in-relation-to-others that become influential entities in both the conscious and unconscious mind. Within this framework, difficulties may arise from disruptions of various sorts during development, most likely the result of the interaction of constitutional factors and environmental conditions. These disruptions may cause the child to internalize relationships as being "bad," leading to maladaptive psychic constructions that are played out to the patient's detriment in current life. *Object relations theory* posits a model of treatment that is based on modifying pathological images of self and others, refining them or replacing them with more helpful and benign internal models and characters.

● ● ●

Although everyone has the need throughout life for a certain amount of affirmation, people with these kinds of problems require excessive ongoing validation and confirmation to maintain any equilibrium.

● ● ●

Because BPD is often related to disturbances of identity and the self, concepts and techniques from *self psychology* may be applicable at times. Originally formulated by Heinz Kohut (1984), and elaborated on by others, this paradigm focuses on the role of an individual's thoughts about the expectations and assessments of others in the shaping and maintenance of self-concept and self-esteem. Some patients depend heavily on certain responses from other people to be able to function. Although everyone has the need throughout life for a certain amount of affirmation, people with these kinds of problems require excessive ongoing validation and confirmation to maintain any equilibrium. As a result, people with such difficulty cannot internally regulate their sense of self and thus may feel as if they are required to be perfect or to perform for others to gain adequate attention. This dynamic for need gratification might be manifested in treatment in the form of a "mirror transference," whereby the patient is compelled to act in various ways to try to gain the therapist's admiration and approval. Patient and therapist may then work together to identify and understand this dynamic to help free the patient from the burden of relying on others for self-esteem maintenance. The self psychology approach, applied to borderline pathology most notably by Adler (e.g., Adler 1993), has been influential in informing therapists about the important role of empathy in helping their patients to develop more cohesive and stable self-identities.

Ego psychology has provided certain ideas that may also be informative in understanding how to work with some of the problems associated with BPD. (The ego is thought to be the part of the psyche that mediates between the external world and the unconscious.) Within the ego psychology model, a system of unconscious defenses was elaborated as ways the mind attempts to help the individual feel comfortable and function effectively while experiencing various psychological pressures (Gabbard 2000). When internal conflict, painful anxiety, or troubling emotions arise that a person may not want to experience, he or she may defend against these internal pressures by thinking, feeling, or acting in unproductive ways. For example, one of the most widely discussed defenses is repression, whereby a painful, traumatic, or undesirable experience or thought is pushed out of conscious awareness. One of the key features of BPD is the use of the *splitting* defense. Individuals who cannot tolerate ambiguity or contradictions because of the emotional turmoil they create instead see the world in black-and-white terms, vacillating between seeing situations or other people as all good or all bad (Gunderson 2001).

This latter phenomenon as part of borderline conditions has been explicated extensively by Kernberg (1967), using elements of object relations theory and ego psychology. According to this formulation, at the root of borderline disturbance are aggressive impulses that constantly threaten to destroy positive internal images of the self and others. Consequently, as the person "splits" his or her mind into pieces to protect the good images from the bad, his or her self-concept becomes fractured— hence the identity problems associated with BPD. This is problematic for the patient and can be a challenge to treatment, because there is often a pattern of alternating idealization and denigration of the therapist. An important goal is to help the patient, over time, to become aware of this pattern, assisting in the further integration of the inner world so that ambivalence and ambiguity can be tolerated.

There are now many psychoanalysts and psychodynamic psychotherapists who are experienced in working successfully with patients with BPD. Careful selection of a therapist should be undertaken with the above-mentioned considerations in mind. There are also specific psycho-analytically informed **manualized treatments** being employed by a select group of clinicians working with BPD. That is, for both research and treatment purposes, written manuals have been developed with directives for clinicians in utilizing the specific psychotherapeutic approach with BPD patients. Several of these treatments are described in the following subsections.

Psychoanalytically Informed Supportive Psychotherapy in BPD

Originally developed for a major study at New York Presbyterian Hospital Personality Disorders Institute comparing different types of psychotherapy for BPD patients, psychoanalytically informed supportive treatment focuses on the identity problems frequently associated with the disorder. A basic assumption is that patients' problematic behaviors and thought processes are attempts at coping with a very fragile sense of self. The goal of this treatment is to help the patient integrate a fractured internal world.

The theoretical mechanism for change posited in this model is the notion that the patient will be able to internalize and identify with a new and positive object and object relationship: the relationship with the therapist. To accomplish this, the therapist works to understand the individual patient's particular conflicts and mental images of others to find ways of intervening in the most helpful fashion. Using a flexible stance in choosing interventions that are the most tolerable to the patient, the therapist seeks to establish a collaborative relationship to promote an increasing collection of positive shared experiences. The therapist uses a moment-to-moment approach to determine what the patient needs at that particular time in trying to maintain a positive atmosphere so the patient can continue to use the treatment productively. This approach also requires that the therapist demonstrate an ongoing warmth and liking toward the patient, even at the patient's worst.

Particular attention is given to helping patients recognize fluctuations in their sense of self (e.g., "When your boyfriend was so angry, it really disrupted your sense of who *you* are") to assist them in learning to deal with these disjunctions. In addition, the therapist makes particular efforts to facilitate and support the patient's experiences of identity (e.g., "Something about that really means a lot to you; let's try to put it into words"). As the patient realizes over time that the therapist recognizes and accepts all the various parts of the patient's psychic world, the patient (it is hoped) will come to value all parts of herself or himself, even those that often may be disowned.

Transference-Focused Psychotherapy

Another manualized approach developed for treatment and research by the Personality Disorders Institute at New York Presbyterian Hospital is transference-focused psychotherapy (TFP) (Yeomans et al. 2002). TFP is a twice-weekly approach that emphasizes a collaboration between the patient and therapist in setting up and maintaining the contract for and structure of treatment—that is, a shared agreement regarding the time, place, and session length of the treatment and conditions for intersession contacts. Because of the challenges often imposed on a treatment by the tumultuous nature of BPD, having this agreed-on structure in place helps the patient and therapist to weather the storms that may occur as the patient's conflicts emerge in the therapy relationship (in the transference).

● ● ●

Transference-focused psychotherapy assumes that the impulsive self-destructive behaviors, chaotic relationships, distorted perceptions, and fragmented identity in BPD stem from splitting that occurs in the person's psyche.

● ● ●

Based on the formulations of Kernberg described above under "Use of Theoretical Models in Treating BPD," the primary theoretical assumption of TFP is that the impulsive self-destructive behaviors, chaotic relationships, distorted perceptions, and fragmented identity associated with BPD stem from splitting that occurs in the person's psyche. Over time, various *object relations dyads,* or images (sometimes distorted) of self-in-relation-to-other, are internalized. Different dyads are linked with different aspects of the self, and there are varying emotion constellations associated with the dyads. Due to a combination of temperamental and environmental factors, these dyads do not exist in an integrated sense in the patient's mind. To protect the good and helpful images from being corrupted and destroyed by the hateful and destructive images—a fundamental fear in this scenario—the inner world is unconsciously split up into various pieces. Although using such means to attempt to preserve whatever internal good there might be is understandable, it is at great expense that this is done. This constant warring of the parts of the self is thought to account for the dramatic behavioral, cognitive, and emotional symptoms of BPD.

As the patient experiences and manifests this turmoil in the therapy relationship, it is the task of TFP to identify the underlying object relations dyads that are at play in the present time, infusing the patient's view of the self and others. By working with the material that emerges in the therapy relationship, the patient and therapist can collaborate in discussing and trying to understand what is occurring in the here and now, to shed light on the underlying dynamics of the patient's psyche. Through both addressing the internalized representations of relationships that color the patient's current functioning and dealing with the strong and painful emotions that accompany them, the therapist seeks to provide the patient with the opportunity to integrate parts of the self so that these parts no longer have to be psychologically warded off or disowned. Thus the therapy relationship is the vehicle for learning about the patient's inner world and for providing a means of change through interpretations in the context of a safe and predictable structure.

Cognitive-Behavioral Therapies: General Description

The cognitive-behavioral tradition, generally speaking, focuses predominantly on observable behaviors and consciously available thoughts. The cognitive aspects derive from the idea that people are information-processing beings who develop their own particular patterns of thinking and interacting as adaptive means of mastering relationships and the environment (Beck 1990). Personality disorders arise when maladaptive responses and disturbed core beliefs are developed, stemming from perceptions and ideas that became distorted as a result of innate sensitivity, early social learning, or (sometimes) traumatic events.

One way of describing how people think is based on their having established somewhat fixed *schemas,* which include intrinsic assumptions about how the world works and how one should respond. Perceptions and reactions then become programmed based on the individual's particular collection of schemas. However, in the case of personality disorders, the long-standing maladaptive schemas lead the person into disturbed cognitive-interpersonal cycles that are self-perpetuating. In most cases, these patterns have become automatic and so are outside of the person's immediate awareness.

The behavior therapy component arises from learning theory, which holds that behaviors are conditioned and reinforced by the environment. Because maladaptive behaviors, like other behaviors, have been learned, according to this model change occurs when the patient is assisted in unlearning problematic tendencies (Wolpe 1995). This is facilitated through the use of techniques such as skills and assertiveness training, systematic desensitization, and relaxation exercises.

Fundamentally, the purpose of cognitive-behavioral therapy is to identify and modify destructive patterns of behaving and thinking. Compared with psychodynamic psychotherapy and psychoanalysis, cognitive-behavioral treatments tend to be shorter in duration and more specifically goal oriented and skills focused, with more directive interventions by the therapist. Because some cognitive-behavioral therapies involve 20 or fewer sessions, they should not be pursued as the sole psychotherapeutic treatment. There is evidence that at least 1 year of intensive treatment is required for any measurable improvement of BPD to occur (American Psychiatric Association 2001). There are several treatment variations from within this paradigm that have been developed specifically for BPD.

Dialectical Behavior Therapy

Dialectical behavior therapy (DBT) was developed by Marsha Linehan predominantly for the treatment of BPD patients experiencing chronic problems with suicide gestures and attempts. It is now perhaps the most widely used cognitive-behavioral therapy for BPD. DBT is a manualized treatment that combines techniques from cognitive, behavioral, and supportive approaches. The goals of the therapy are to reduce life-threatening behaviors, address behaviors that interfere with the treatment process itself, and modify behaviors that significantly impair the patient's quality of life.

● ● ●

Within the DBT paradigm, the nature of BPD is thought to revolve around impaired regulation of emotions, stemming from biological sensitivity interacting with an early environment lacking in emotional validation.

● ● ●

Within the DBT paradigm, the nature of BPD is thought to revolve around impaired regulation of emotions, stemming from biological sensitivity interacting with an early environment lacking in emotional validation. Linehan (1993a) used the term *dialectics* to describe a therapeutic approach that strives to reconcile opposites in the context of pursuing a process of synthesis. Understood in the broadest terms, this concept means that treatment must provide an environment that accepts the ways patients currently are while also trying to help them change ("radical acceptance"). That is, the therapist validates the patient's experiences and at the same time uses problem solving in an effort to modify maladaptive thinking patterns and teach new ways of coping. Although the therapy relationship is considered central as the laboratory for change, at times it is also the only thing that is keeping seriously suicidal patients alive.

Within DBT, treatment planning proceeds from eight basic assumptions (Linehan 1993a): 1) patients are doing the best they can; 2) patients want to improve; 3) patients need to do better, try harder, and be more motivated to change; 4) patients may not have caused all of their own problems, but they have to solve them anyway; 5) the lives of suicidal borderline individuals are unbearable as they are currently being lived; 6) patients must learn new behaviors in all relevant contexts; 7) patients cannot fail in therapy; 8) therapists treating borderline patients need support.

In joining a DBT program, patients participate in both weekly individual therapy and weekly group skills training for 1 year (Linehan 1993a). The individual psychotherapy is the core of the program, and the individual therapist is the primary clinician on the team responsible for the patient. Because this aspect of the treatment serves as the foundation for all ongoing work, patients are required to be in individual therapy as a prerequisite for participating in other aspects of DBT. Working with the individual therapist is also quite crucial in helping the patient to integrate what is learned in the group components of the experience. Individual therapists are accessible by telephone between sessions, and the lengths of therapy sessions vary according to the needs of the patient at a particular time.

Using the manual prepared specifically for this purpose (Linehan 1993b), the group skills training program is conducted in a psychoeducational format employing practice exercises, handouts, and homework sheets. The groups target core mindfulness, interpersonal effectiveness, distress tolerance, and emotional regulation issues. The main goal is to help the patient acquire a new repertoire of responses and learn to apply these responses in relevant situations. A very active approach is taken by therapists to ensure that the patients are also actively engaging in the training in a productive way. After completing the skills training group, individuals may join optional supportive process groups available to them on an ongoing basis.

Schema Therapy for BPD

Jeffrey Young and his colleagues (Bricker et al. 1993) formulated the concept of an early maladaptive schema, defined as "a long-standing and pervasive theme that originates in childhood; defines the individual's behaviors, thoughts, feelings, and relationships with other people; and leads to maladaptive consequences" (p. 89). Maladaptive schemas arise as deeply entrenched patterns of response, developed in early in life, as means of trying to organize experience of self and others in a world that may have been filled with neglect, instability, or abuse. Although they serve as logical solutions in childhood, the schemas continue to organize the individual in adulthood, when they are ineffective ways of trying to meet basic needs and become associated with negative emotions and impaired functioning. The goal of schema-focused therapy is to help patients identify distortions in thinking and challenge underlying beliefs that routinely result in problems of living.

Eighteen types of schemas falling into three domains—instability and disconnection, impaired autonomy, and undesirability—were originally identified (Bricker et al. 1993). For example, one might hold to a predominant maladaptive schema centered on the fear of being abandoned, which would result in excessive jealousy and clinging in relationships; therapy would center on modifying this outlook. However, in their work with patients with BPD, the team realized that these patients almost always have most of the 18 schemas, particularly abandonment, mistrust/abuse, emotional deprivation, defectiveness, insufficient self-control, subjugation, and punitiveness (Young et al. 2003). Furthermore, because BPD is associated with rapidly shifting moods and states of mind, it became a challenge to concentrate work on one or two specific types of schemas that are seen as stable sets of traits. Consequently, five main modes were identified as pertaining to BPD patients: "abandoned child," "angry and impulsive child," "punitive parent," "detached protector," and "healthy adult."

A major therapeutic goal of this approach as applied to BPD is to greatly enhance the "healthy adult" mode of the patient's functioning. In the actual course of treatment, the therapist learns how to track the individual's various modes in session and utilize strategies appropriate to each one of the modes. For example, in "abandoned child" mode, the therapist tries to satisfy many of the patient's unmet childhood needs for safety, caring, autonomy, and self-expression. Through empathy and nurturing, the therapist aims to re-parent the patient within appropriate therapeutic limits. At different times throughout the treatment, cognitive-behavioral techniques such as guided imagery, education, assertiveness training, and role playing may be used.

STEPPS Group Treatment Program for BPD

Begun in 1995 at the University of Iowa, Systems Training for Emotional Predictability and Problem Solving (STEPPS) involves two phases of treatment: 1) a basic skills group that meets for 20 weeks and; 2) a 1-year, twice-monthly advanced group program called STAIRWAYS—for Setting goals, Trusting and taking risks, Anger management, Impulsivity control, Relationship behavior, Writing a script, Assertiveness training, Your journey, and Schemas revisited (Blum et al. 2002). This program was developed specifically as a means for reducing self-harm behaviors and psychiatric hospitalization rates, and it can be used as an adjunct to other ongoing psychotherapeutic treatments. In addition, the brief nature of the model is partly a reflection of the geographic context from which it arose; that is, Iowa is a rural state where many patients need to drive long distances for treatment. The STEPPS team also desired to create an approach that practitioners could easily utilize without having to engage in extensive special training.

● ● ●

The STEPPS approach rests on the assumption that BPD patients have defects in their ability to regulate the intensity of emotions.

● ● ●

The STEPPS approach rests on the assumption that BPD patients have defects in their ability to regulate the intensity of emotions. In fact, an alternative term to BPD used in this context is *emotional intensity disorder* (Blum et al. 2002). First, through a three-step cognitive-behavioral skills training approach, patients are taught about the feelings and behaviors associated with BPD and that change is possible. Second, there is a sequence on emotion management training, highlighting specific skills for recognizing schemas and trigger situations and strategies for responding. The third component centers on behavior management training, reviewing such skills as goal setting, relaxation activities, and avoiding abusive behaviors as means of responding in various functional areas of life when emotions threaten to overwhelm the patient's ability to cope.

An important aspect of this treatment is the systems component, which involves the participation of family members and significant others, known as the reinforcement team. Through specific sessions designed for the reinforcement team, team members are educated about

BPD and the content of the STEPPS program. In addition, they are taught about ways of responding to the BPD patient that are consistent and that reinforce what the patient is learning in the group.

Empirical Evidence for the Effectiveness of Psychotherapies in BPD

A variety of research efforts studying psychotherapy for BPD have been conducted over the years using disparate methodological approaches; several notable studies are summarized here. Stevenson and Meares (1992) demonstrated significant improvement in a group of 30 borderline patients who were treated for 12 months with twice-weekly psychodynamic psychotherapy. Bateman and Fonagy (1999) assessed the progress of a group of 38 patients with BPD who either 1) were treated for 18 months in individual and group psychoanalytic psychotherapy as part of a partial hospitalization program or 2) received standard psychiatric treatment. Patients in the psychoanalytic psychotherapy program showed significantly greater improvements than those in the comparison group on measures of depression, interpersonal function, number of suicide attempts and self-harm, and inpatient admissions. Improvement for this group started as early as 6 months into treatment and continued through the 18-month period. In addition, a follow-up study by the same authors (Bateman and Fonagy 2001) showed that the patients who were treated in the psychodynamic partial hospitalization program not only maintained their gains but also continued to show improvement over an 18-month follow-up period, whereas those receiving standard psychiatric treatment showed only limited changes over the same period.

● ● ●

By the end of 1 year of treatment, the patients receiving DBT had less parasuicidal behavior and had spent fewer days in the hospital than those in the comparison group.

● ● ●

Linehan and colleagues (1991) conducted a study comparing two groups of patients with BPD having symptoms of self-harm (parasuicidal), with one group receiving DBT and the other receiving treatment as usual. By the end of 1 year of treatment, the patients in the DBT group had less parasuicidal behavior and had spent fewer days in the hospital than those in the comparison group. The DBT patients also showed a greater capacity for staying in treatment with the same therapist. A post-treatment follow-up study (Linehan et al. 1993) showed that after 1 year the improvement in self-harm behavior of the DBT group did not persist, but there were fewer hospital days for this group during the period. An additional study (Linehan et al. 1999) applying DBT to a group of patients with BPD and drug dependence showed some promise that DBT can be helpful in reducing drug use in this population.

It should be noted that the groups used in these various studies have been rather small, arising from the difficult patient population and the resource-intensive nature of this kind of research. In this era of scarce funding for such studies it is clear that additional research is needed in assessing various psychotherapeutic approaches. Several studies are currently being conducted by the New York State Psychiatric Institute (on DBT and supportive therapy groups) and New York Presbyterian Personality Disorders Institute (on TFP, DBT, and supportive therapy groups). It is to be hoped that these studies will yield informative results in the near future.

Several recent reviews have summarized the results of empirical studies testing the efficacy or effectiveness of various psychotherapeutic approaches for BPD (American Psychiatric Association 2001; Gabbard 2000; Gunderson 2001; Perry and Bond 2000), and the reader is referred to these sources for additional details. It must be noted, however, that the authors of the various reviews were all optimistic about the prospects for BPD patients improving in treatment. Gabbard (2000) concluded that studies of psychodynamic psychotherapy demonstrate "that although there is no 'quick fix' for BPD, those patients who stay in dynamic therapy for a substantial period of time may experience significant improvement" (p. 433). Furthermore, Gabbard noted empirical evidence for the cost-effectiveness of supporting long-term psychodynamic outpatient therapy and DBT for borderline patients, which results in decreased use of psychiatric hospitals and other general medical treatments. Perry and Bond (2000) summarized their review of the literature this way: "Despite the caveats about the limitations of the existing studies, our current level of knowledge is sufficient to warrant a message of hope" (p. 27).

Conclusion

With the recent adoption of the American Psychiatric Association's "Practice Guideline for the Treatment of Patients With Borderline Personality Disorder" (American Psychiatric Association 2001), the psychiatric establishment has officially underscored the pressing need for the mental health field to directly address issues related to borderline personality. BPD represents a particular set of complicated and often debilitating challenges, apart from other disorders, and warrants special consideration in the formulation of treatment approaches. As outlined in this chapter, there are a growing number of therapies and therapists who are well prepared to engage in assisting patients with BPD in improving their lives. Moreover, clinical experience and increasing evidence in the empirical literature have shown that with proper treatment and time invested, a large majority of these patients can do quite well.

What Families Need to Know

Key Messages in This Chapter

- Most people with BPD will benefit from extended psychotherapy to help them with their overall functioning.
- Although early attempts to use classical psychoanalysis in individuals with borderline issues proved unsuccessful, modified versions of this form of treatment work well with many patients.
- Several forms of psychodynamic psychotherapies, based on psychoanalytic theory, help the person with BPD work to identify patterns of thoughts, emotions, and behaviors that may not be conscious. The relationship with the therapist is the primary vehicle for change.
- Cognitive-behavioral therapies involve attempts to identify and modify destructive patterns of thinking and behaving through skills training. These therapies are shorter in duration than psychodynamic psychotherapies and involve more direct interventions by the therapist.
- The alliance established with the therapist is essential to the success of all types of psychotherapy used for BPD. A key element in all forms of therapy is the ongoing support of the patient.
- Regardless of the form of psychotherapy chosen, the first priority is to ensure that the person with BPD is not in danger of harming himself or herself. Medications and other programs (such as treatment for substance abuse) may be necessary at the same time (adjunctively).
- Several small studies have demonstrated the success of various forms of psychotherapy in reducing parasuicidal behavior, drug dependence, and time spent in the hospital for some groups of patients with BPD. With proper treatment over an extended period of time, many patients can do quite well.

Key Words in This Chapter

adjunctive   added to or joined with other treatments.

alliance   a relationship between patient and therapist that fosters trust and facilitates successful treatment.

cognitive-behavioral therapies   therapies focusing on thoughts, feelings, and actions the person is aware of; treatment is aimed at using the thinking process to reframe, restructure, and solve problems.

constellation   a collection or assemblage (of symptoms).

ego psychology   psychological paradigm focusing on the organizing activity of the mind that uses unconscious defense mechanisms (e.g., repression, denial) to function in the world.

manualized treatments   treatments based on written manuals containing specific directions for the therapist, for example, dialectical behavior therapy (DBT); these approaches allow treatments to be replicated and research to be standardized.

neurotic   having a chronic or recurrent nonpsychotic disorder characterized mainly by anxiety.

nomenclature   a system of technical or scientific names.

object relations theory   the belief that early experiences of the self in relationship to other people (objects) shape the way one relates to others as an adult.

psychodynamic psychotherapies   therapies focusing on thoughts and feelings that the patient may not be consciously aware of.

psychotic   exhibiting a loss of reality testing and impairment of mental, social, and personal functioning.

schemas   fixed ideas, beliefs, or assumptions about self, others, or the way the world works, often arising in childhood.

self psychology   psychological paradigm emphasizing the importance of validation and empathy from others in maintaining self-esteem.

splitting   a defense mechanism whereby, to control emotional turmoil or avoid inner conflicts, a person views the world in black-and-white terms and sees people as all good or all bad.

transference   old wishes, expectations, and conflicts that shape present relationships and come to light in the relationship with the therapist.

References

Adler G: The psychotherapy of core borderline psychopathology. Am J Psychother 47:194–205, 1993

American Psychiatric Association: Practice Guideline for the Treatment of Patients With Borderline Personality Disorder. Washington, DC, American Psychiatric Association, 2001

Bach S: On treating the difficult patient, in The Modern Freudians. Edited by Ellman CS, Grand S, Silvan M, et al. Northvale, NJ, Jason Aronson, 1998, pp 185–195

Bateman A, Fonagy P: Effectiveness of partial hospitalization in the treatment of borderline personality disorder: a randomized controlled trial. Am J Psychiatry 156:1563–1569, 1999

Bateman A, Fonagy P: Treatment of borderline personality disorder with psychoanalytically oriented partial hospitalization: an 18-month follow-up. Am J Psychiatry 158:36–42, 2001

Beck AT, Freeman A: Cognitive Therapy of Personality Disorders. New York, Guilford, 1990

Blum N, Pfohl B, St. John D, et al: STEPPS: a cognitive-behavioral systems-based group treatment for outpatients with borderline personality disorder—a preliminary report. Compr Psychiatry 43:301–310, 2002

Bricker D, Young JE, Flanagan CM: Schema-focused cognitive therapy: a comprehensive framework for characterological problems, in Cognitive Therapies in Action. Edited by Kuehlwein KT, Rosen H. San Francisco, CA, Jossey-Bass, 1993, pp 88–125

Gabbard GO: Psychodynamic Psychiatry in Clinical Practice. Washington, DC, American Psychiatric Press, 2000

Gunderson JG: Borderline Personality Disorder: A Clinical Guide. Washington, DC, American Psychiatric Publishing, 2001

Kernberg OF: Borderline personality organization. J Am Psychoanal Assoc 15:641–685, 1967

Kernberg OF: Borderline Conditions and Pathological Narcissism. New York, Jason Aronson, 1975

Kernberg OF: Technical considerations in the treatment of borderline personality organization. J Am Psychoanal Assoc 24:795–829, 1976

Knight RP: Borderline states (1953), in Current and Historical Perspectives on the Borderline Patient. Edited by Fine R. New York, Brunner/Mazel, 1989, pp 96–108

Kohut H: How Does Analysis Cure? Chicago, IL, University of Chicago Press, 1984

Linehan MM: Cognitive-Behavioral Treatment of Borderline Personality Disorder. New York, Guilford, 1993a

Linehan MM: Skills Training Manual for Treating Borderline Personality Disorder. New York, Guilford, 1993b

Linehan MM, Armstrong HE, Suarez A, et al: Cognitive-behavioral treatment of chronically parasuicidal borderline patients. Arch Gen Psychiatry 48:1060–1064, 1991

Linehan MM, Heard HL, Armstrong HE: Naturalistic follow-up of a behavioral treatment for chronically parasuicidal borderline patients. Arch Gen Psychiatry 50:971–974, 1993

Linehan MM, Schmidt H III, Dimeff LA, et al: Dialectical behavior therapy for patients with borderline personality disorder and drug-dependence. Am J Addict 8:279–292, 1999

Perry JC, Bond M: Empirical studies of psychotherapy for personality disorders, in Psychotherapy for Personality Disorders (Review of Psychiatry, Vol 19; Oldham JM, Riba MB, series eds). Edited by Gunderson JG, Gabbard GO. Washington, DC, American Psychiatric Press, 2000, pp 1–31

Pine F: Drive, Ego, Object, and Self. New York, Basic Books, 1990

Stevenson J, Meares R: An outcome study of psychotherapy for patients with borderline personality disorder. Am J Psychiatry 149:358–362, 1992

Stone L: The widening scope of indications for psychoanalysis. J Am Psychoanal Assoc 2:567–594, 1954

Stone MH: The borderline syndrome: evolution of the term, genetic aspects, and prognosis. Am J Psychother 31:345–365, 1977

Winston A, Rosenthal RN, Muran JC: Supportive psychotherapy, in Handbook of Personality Disorders. Edited by Livesley WJ. New York, Guilford, 2001, pp 344–358

Wolpe J: Reciprocal inhibition: major agent of behavior change, in Theories of Behavior Change. Edited by O'Donohue W, Krasner L. Washington, DC, American Psychological Association, 1995, pp 23–57

Yeomans FE, Clarkin JF, Kernberg OF: A Primer of Transference-Focused Psychotherapy for the Borderline Patient. Northvale, NJ, Jason Aronson, 2002

Young J, Klosko J, Weishaar M: Schema therapy for borderline personality disorder, in Schema Therapy: A Practitioner's Guide. New York, Guilford, 2003, pp 306–372

• 3 •

Suicidal and Self-Injurious Behavior in Borderline Personality Disorder

A Self-Regulation Model

Barbara Stanley, Ph.D.
Beth S. Brodsky, Ph.D.

Deliberately inflicted self-harm in the context of borderline personality disorder (BPD) can be disturbing, frightening, and shame provoking to individuals who engage in it, to their families, and to the clinicians who care for them. This behavior is particularly confusing because of its seemingly paradoxical nature. On one hand, it causes extraordinary physical and emotional suffering. On the other hand, the behavior is often designed for and experienced as relieving suffering. Many individuals who commit self-harm describe it as substituting physical suffering, which is easier to tolerate and plainly visible, for emotional pain and suffering, which is experienced as intolerable and is mostly invisible to others. Also, individuals get confused about whether their emotional suffering is real or not. Physical damage provides concrete proof of emotional suffering. Patients often report, "Only someone who is deeply distressed would inflict this kind of self-harm." The physical pain also provides justification, after the fact, for their negative emotional state. Another aspect of this seeming paradox is that although the behavior causes physical damage to individuals, it can also function as a compromise solution that permits them to go on living. Patients think, "If I cut myself or take this relatively small overdose, I won't have to really kill myself." Thus, although clinicians may react to self-harm by hospitalizing the self-injurer, it may be unnecessary and even counterproductive to take this action if the behavior has already given the individual "permission" to go on living. This may be true not just for nonsuicidal self-injury but also for low-lethality suicide attempts. There is a tendency on the part of professionals and family members to ascribe suicidal intent to nonsuicidal self-injury, such as superficial cutting. This can result in unnecessary hospitalization and disruption of the individual's functioning, leading to loss of work or school dismissal and fear, anger, or withdrawal by family members and friends (Gunderson and Ridolfi 2001). This misjudgment and misunderstanding is related to another paradoxical aspect of self-harm in the context of BPD: both an underappreciation of and an overreaction to suicidality.

● ● ●

Many who commit self-harm describe it as substituting physical suffering for emotional pain and suffering, which is experienced as intolerable and is mostly invisible to others.

● ● ●

Many individuals with BPD experience frequent nonsuicidal self-injury along with chronic **suicidal ideation,** suicide threats, and intermittent nonlethal suicide attempts. This makes prediction of actual suicide risk very difficult (Fine and Sansone 1990). Although there can be a tendency to hospitalize when it is not **clinically** indicated, professionals and family members can develop a "boy who cried wolf" reaction to repeated low-lethality suicide attempts, nonsuicidal self-injury, and chronic suicidal ideation. In this scenario, clinicians and family members can become almost immune to concern about the individual's self-injury and suicidality after repeated episodes accompanied by chronic suicidal ideation and urges. These caregivers can become complacent, underestimating or neglecting genuine suicide risk, and this may contribute to a high rate of suicide completion. In fact, the population of individuals with BPD is at high risk for completed suicide, with a lifetime suicide rate of about 9%–10%. Relatedly, the low medical lethality and seemingly minor precipitants for many self-injury episodes may contribute to the misperception that self-injury is merely manipulative and attention seeking and is thus not to be taken seriously (Leibenluft et al. 1987). Therefore, although suicidal behavior occurs in the context of many psychiatric disorders, the combination of nonlethal self-injury, such as superficial cutting and burning, together with multiple low-lethality suicide attempts, is an almost exclusive phenomenon of BPD. Its high incidence in BPD presents a formidable challenge to helping individuals with this problem. In fact, some clinicians refuse to treat patients with BPD because of the sense of burden, confusion, stress, and liability in working with such high-risk patients. This is an unfortunate circumstance. Although treating individuals with BPD can be stressful, as is any clinical work with patients who have life-threatening illness, it can also be an extremely rewarding and productive experience. Patients can rid themselves of chronic suicidal ideation and eliminate self-injurious behavior as a means of coping.

● ● ●

Although treating people with BPD can be stressful, as is any clinical work with patients who have life-threatening illness, it can also be an extremely rewarding and productive experience.

● ● ●

The purpose of this chapter is to provide a comprehensive review, from both clinical and *empirical* perspectives, of what is currently known about the emotional and physical experience of individuals with BPD who intentionally harm themselves, either as suicide attempts or as nonsuicidal self-injury.

We discuss the following areas:

- The definition of relevant terms and the experience of self-injury, including its function and purpose, its precipitants, the vulnerabilities that increase its likelihood, and it aftereffects
- The distinction between suicidal behavior and nonsuicidal self-harm and the ways in which they sometimes overlap
- Speculation as to how the experience of suicidality in individuals with BPD may differ from suicidal behavior in depressed individuals
- Description of clinical approaches to investigating the nature of self-injury and to helping individuals handle urges to attempt suicide and to self-injure
- Development of a new model: the self-regulation action model of suicidal behavior and nonsuicidal self-injury in individuals with BPD

- Illustration, using clinical examples, of how this understanding can be clinically applied toward more effective treatment
- Recommendations for future research

In this chapter we focus primarily on the psychological factors related to the experience of self-injury. However, when findings are relevant to the *phenomenology* of self-injury we also discuss recent advances in the understanding of the neurobiological systems that may be implicated in self-injurious behavior.

Background and Definitions

Despite recent clinical and media attention to self-injurious behavior, not enough is understood regarding the actual experience of individuals who intentionally injure themselves without causing lethal harm. Even the terms and their definitions are unclear and conflicting. Several terms that have been used to discuss self-directed harm need to be clarified.

● ● ●

Deliberate self-harm includes two forms of self-destructive behavior: one with an intent to die and one in which the self-inflicted damage does not connote this intent.

● ● ●

Deliberate self-harm includes two forms of self-destructive behavior: one with an intent to die and one in which the self-inflicted damage does not connote this intent. Both forms involve self-inflicted physical harm but do not include behaviors in which individuals provoke others into harming them, such as getting into fights. The two types of self-harm discussed here are defined as follows:

1. **Suicide attempt:** A suicide attempt is defined as an intentionally self-destructive act performed with at least partial intent to die. Although this is an apparently straightforward definition, the assessment of an individual's subjective intent is challenging for a number of reasons. Intent may be difficult to determine through direct inquiry, because retrospective reports can be influenced by reinterpretation and by outcome and may no longer be accurate descriptions of the individual's state of mind at the time of the self-injury. Clinically, suicidal intent is often deduced by external behaviors or factors (such as how

medically lethal the self-injury is) or by the circumstances (such as the likelihood of being discovered during or immediately after the act surrounding the self-injury). These deductions can lead to erroneous assumptions, particularly for individuals with BPD who self-injure for many reasons and in whom the intent to die is often ambiguous. Perception of intent can also be distorted by the existence of previous nonlethal attempts (Stanley et al. 2001).

2. **Self-injurious behavior:** Nonsuicidal self-injury, sometimes called *self-mutilation,* is defined as intentional self-destructive behavior performed with no intent to die. Such self-injury with no suicidal intent is quite particular to the BPD diagnosis and can be understood within the context of BPD **pathology** as an effort to regulate emotions. Although suicidal intent is often ascribed to these behaviors by clinicians and family members, individuals with BPD are often quite clear that their intent is quite to the contrary and that these behaviors are often used in an attempt to feel better.

Two other terms are important to mention: self-mutilation and **para-suicide.** Although the term *self-mutilation* is commonly used to describe nonsuicidal self-harm, we believe that it is not inclusive enough. Some forms of self-injury, such as cutting and burning, involve mutilation; others, such as head banging and hitting oneself, do not. The term *parasuicide* is often used incorrectly. Although the term is mistakenly thought to include only behaviors without suicide intent, its actual definition is *any* self-injurious behavior, with or without suicidal intent, that does not result in death. Thus all suicide attempts fall into the category of parasuicide, as do self-mutilation and nonsuicidal self-injury.

Prevalence and Significance of the Problem

As stated earlier, individuals with BPD have approximately a 9%–10% lifetime rate of suicide (Linehan et al. 1991; Stone et al. 1987a, 1987b; Ventura et al. 1997). It is estimated that up to 75% of individuals with BPD have made nonlethal suicide attempts (Fyer 1988; Gunderson 1984), with nearly 50% making at least one severe attempt (Fyer 1988). Furthermore, approximately 80% of hospitalized patients with BPD have engaged in self-mutilation—usually cutting, burning the skin, or hitting themselves without the intention to die (Shearer et al. 1988). Although these figures are strikingly high, they may somewhat overestimate the incidence of these behaviors in the overall BPD population, because the data were derived largely from studies of hospitalized patients. Self-mutilation itself is a risk factor for suicidal behavior, as 55%–85% of self-mutilators have made at least one suicide attempt (Favazza and Conterio 1989; Gardner and Gardner 1975; Rosenthal et al. 1972; Roy 1978). The combination of suicidal behavior and self-mutilation is especially common in BPD (Soloff et al. 1994).

Although suicide attempts and nonsuicidal self-injury are both self-destructive, they are usually quite distinct in the individual's mind and are very different in intent and method. The medical lethality of these two types of behavior may be similar, owing to miscalculations and distortions of the perception of lethality of a given act. Stanley et al. (2001) found that individuals with BPD who both self-mutilate and make suicide attempts tend to perceive their suicide attempts as less lethal than they actually are, with a greater likelihood of rescue and with less certainty of death. Therefore, ambivalence of suicidal intent interacting with past experience of nonsuicidal self-injury does not necessarily reduce the medical lethality of these suicide attempts. The usual method of suicide attempt in BPD is overdosing (Stanley et al. 2001). Although overdosing is less violent than some methods and is more amenable to low-lethality attempts, this does not necessarily imply less intent to die. A study of method choice, intent, and gender in completed suicide showed that although women who commit suicide use less violent methods (overdoses and carbon monoxide poisoning) than men (guns and hanging), there was no difference in their intent (Denning et al. 2000).

The usual types of nonsuicidal self-injury are cutting the skin (often on the inside of the arms) and burning the skin (arms, legs, and stomach). Also common are self-hitting, head banging, self-burning, self-biting, hair pulling, and skin picking. Shearer's (1994) report of the phenomenology of self-injury documented that the most frequent type of nonsuicidal self-injury among BPD inpatients was superficial cutting or scratching (80%), followed by hitting (24%), burning (20%), and head banging (15%).

Self-Injurious Behavior: Reasons and Functions

A common belief is that nonsuicidal self-injury is attention seeking and manipulative. However, there is both clinical and empirical evidence arguing against this notion. Nonsuicidal self-injury is usually an extremely private behavior; it is often denied and hidden. Individuals who self-injure are often deeply ashamed of their self-injury. Shearer (1994) and Brodsky et al. (1995) independently reported that approximately 50% of BPD inpatients hide the fact that they self-injure and do not let anyone know about it. Suyemoto (1998) reports that isolation from others almost always precedes the actual act of self-mutilation.

• • •

Nonsuicidal self-injury is usually an extremely private behavior; it is often denied and hidden. People who self-injure are often deeply ashamed of their self-injury.

• • •

Nevertheless, people feel manipulated by self-injury, and it does draw attention. It is important to distinguish between intent and effect. Suyemoto (1998) made the point that self-mutilators, feeling overwhelmed by their emotions, are often unaware of the effect they have on others. However, the attention that results from self-mutilation can become reinforcing, so that even when the behavior was originally intended for purposes of *affect regulation,* the attention that results often becomes a desired consequence. The following are the functions of self-injury that are most commonly reported by patients:

1. **Affect regulation.** Nonsuicidal self-injury appears to make the individual feel better by reducing emotional tension, which is usually experienced as extreme distress, anxiety, anger, guilt, or shame (Favazza and Conterio 1989).
2. **Distraction.** Self-injury is also employed as a distraction from emotional pain. In a manner similar to bulimia with all its rituals and preoccupation, episodes of self-injury can be just as self-absorbing. As such, self-injury becomes an activity that is very engaging and therefore serves as a distraction from distressing emotions and events.
3. **Self-punishment.** Gunderson and Ridolfi (2001) reported from their clinical experience that cutting mostly serves the function of self-punishment, "providing relief from a poorly articulated but intolerable state involving intense shame, remorse, and convictions of badness and alienation" (p. 63).
4. **Concrete proof of emotional distress.** This is mostly for the patient's own benefit and not to provide proof to others. It is difficult for these individuals to believe how terrible they are feeling without visible evidence. Linehan (1993) described the process of *self-invalidation* that occurs in BPD, whereby individuals believe that they are overreacting or that they have no reason to be feeling the way they do, and therefore they are not and should not be feeling that way. A scar or bruise can provide the concrete evidence of their emotional state.

5. **Exertion of control.** Individuals with BPD have great difficulty with affect regulation and therefore often feel out of control. To feel that they are in control of events and emotions, they self-injure. By harming themselves, they are taking control of the out-of-control behaviors of others or of the external events that cause their distress (Favazza 1989).

6. **Alleviation of numbness and depersonalization.** Favazza (1989) calls this function "return to reality." Many individuals with BPD experience very distressing feelings in response to upsetting events, interactions, or emotions. These feelings can become overwhelming and can lead to a sense of being on "emotional overload." It is very painful to remain in this state, and as a result patients can enter a state of numbness and *depersonalization.* However, this state is also disconcerting and is hard to snap out of. Self-injury is one of the few behaviors that help to alleviate this numbness.

7. **Ventilation of anger.** Acting on angry feelings through self-harm seems safer and less guilt producing than to express anger toward others (Favazza 1989).

Among a sample of inpatients with BPD (Shearer 1994), the most frequently reported functions of nonsuicidal self-injury were as follows: to feel concrete pain instead of overwhelming emotional pain (59%), to inflict self-punishment (49%), to reduce anxiety and feelings of despair (39%), to feel in control (22%), to express anger (22%), to feel something when feeling numb or out of touch (20%), to seek help from others (17%), and to keep bad memories away (15%).

The Experience of Self-Injury

There is typically a process leading to self-injury. Some upset—an event, a trigger in the environment—takes place. Gunderson and Ridolfi (2001), Suyemoto (1998), and Russ (1992) emphasized that the trigger is almost always a real or perceived interpersonal loss through separation or abandonment. An interpretation (*cognition*) of the event follows, which usually involves the individual's self-blame or self-condemnation. Emotions escalate, cloud judgment, feel all-consuming, and become *dysregulated,* usually turning into some form of self-hatred. Suyemoto (1998) emphasized that the overwhelming emotion often, but not always, leads to a dissociative response in which the individual goes from feeling intense pain to feeling nothing other than the experience of numbness. Either the painful feelings or the numbness begin to be experienced as a rising internal pressure that becomes difficult to resist. The individual self-injures and experiences an immediate sense of relief from the pressure (Gardner and Cowdry 1985) and a reinstatement of emotional equilibrium.

● ● ●

The trigger for self-injury is almost always a real or perceived interpersonal loss through separation or abandonment.

● ● ●

It is not clear exactly what happens that leads to the sense of relief. Some individuals report that they stop the self-injury when they begin to feel pain. Others stop when they see the blood, as if this is experienced as the release of the tension or the "letting out" of the bad feelings. Leibenluft et al. (1987) made the point that self-injury is remarkably effective in relieving the dysphoric state. Although the relief may be associated with psychological factors such as relief of guilt through self-punishment, Leibenluft and colleagues also acknowledged the possibility of a physiological mechanism such as the relief of one type of pain by inducing a counter-stimulus. They also suggested that perhaps the self-injury stimulates the release of a pain-reducing biochemical agent such as an endorphin. A study by Stanley et al. (2003) indicating the presence of altered concentrations of *endogenous opioids* in the cerebrospinal fluid of self-injurers favors this latter explanation.

Cognitions and Cognitive Factors

The functions of self-injury are very much affected by the cognitions that accompany the emotional experience. Individuals who self-injure often hold fixed beliefs—referred to by Linehan (1993) as "myths" and labeled by J.S. Beck (1995) as "distorted cognitions"—that support the function of the self-injury. For example, individuals with BPD often assume that they cannot handle emotional pain and that physical pain is more tolerable. They believe that they can rid themselves of negative emotions and that self-injury is the only way they can obtain immediate relief from their intolerable emotional states. They believe that by injuring themselves they are more in control than if they were to allow themselves to experience their dysregulated emotions, which they perceive as either coming out of nowhere or triggered by events that they perceive (not always correctly) to be completely out of their control. Individuals who utilize self-injury as an expression of anger believe that it is better to hurt themselves than to express anger, and they believe that it is "wrong" to express angry feelings toward others, particularly people they care about. Those who need to self-punish often believe that they deserve to suffer. There is a need for further research to document these beliefs empirically and to understand how they contribute to self-injury.

● ● ●

People with BPD often assume that they cannot handle emotional pain and that physical pain is more tolerable.

● ● ●

Dissociation, Self-Injurious Behavior, and the Experience of Pain

A few reports (Kemperman et al. 1997; Russ et al. 1993) documented that individuals with BPD who self-injure fall into two distinct groups related to whether or not they experience pain when they self-injure. According to Russ et al. (1993), individuals who do not experience pain during self-injury represent a more impaired population characterized by higher levels of depression, anxiety, impulsivity, *dissociation,* trauma symptoms, number of past suicide attempts, and prevalence of sexual abuse. Kemperman et al. (1997) reported that female patients with BPD who do not experience pain during self-injury discriminate more poorly between noxious thermal stimuli of similar intensity. They conclude that *analgesia* during self-injury is related to both neurosensory and psychological factors.

Neurobiology and Neurocognitive Factors

Neurobiological findings regarding the role of endogenous opioids and serotonergic functioning point to their possible role in suicidal and nonsuicidal self-injury (Winchel and Stanley 1991). *Serotonin* has been implicated in suicide, suicide attempts, impulsivity, and aggression. Although it is known that suicide attempters have altered serotonergic functioning and show higher levels of impulsivity and aggression, it is not clear how this affects the actual self-injury experience. Neuropsychological studies are now under way to investigate the relationship between lower serotonin concentration, impulsivity, and cognitive processes that might affect self-injury. For example, Keilp et al. (2001) identified an impairment in *executive functioning*, beyond that typically found in major depression, among depressed patients who have made a previous high-lethality suicide attempt.

With regard to neuroendocrine functioning in self-injury, in a German case reported by Sachsse and colleagues (2002) it was found that episodes of self-mutilation occurred in response to hyperactivity of the central stress-sensitive *neuroendocrine systems* and increased cortisol secretion. These findings suggest a possible biological basis for the clinical observations that self-mutilation occurs in response to increases in emotional arousal. Stanley et al. (2003) found that concentrations of endogenous opioids were altered in the cerebrospinal fluid of individuals who self-injure. This finding indicates that there may be some central deficit in pain perception or regulation in those who self-injure. Taken together, these findings point to a biological underpinning for all forms of self-injurious behavior.

The Conventional Model of Suicidal Behavior

There is reason to believe that the way psychiatrists have been trained to think about the causes of suicidal behavior, the way the media portray suicide, and the pattern of thinking and acting leading to a suicide attempt do not usually apply to the suicidal individual who also has BPD. Many clinicians and laypersons have a conceptual model of suicidal behavior—that is, what the suicidal person is like and what causes someone to become suicidal—that is based on major depression as the most important contributing factor. In this model, the depressed individual goes through a protracted period of depressed mood, hopelessness, withdrawal, and isolation. Often this depression is preceded by some form of psychosocial stressor, usually a significant loss. Depression can culminate in a feeling that life is not worth living and may lead to a suicide attempt. After the attempt, the individual typically feels upset if the attempt was not "successful" (i.e., did not result in death).

● ● ●

The model of suicidal behavior based on major depression often does not seem to apply to suicide attempts by people with BPD.

● ● ●

This conventional model of suicidal behavior often does not seem to apply to suicide attempts by persons with BPD. Another confusing aspect of the clinical picture is that individuals with BPD often describe suicide attempts in the same way that they describe self-injury episodes. Suicide attempts by individuals with BPD may also serve an emotion-regulation function similar to that of self-injury episodes, because the individuals tend to feel better after making a suicide attempt.

We present two case illustrations that demonstrate how the conventional understanding of suicidality is inadequate in explaining the suicidal states of many individuals with BPD.

Case Example 1

CB is a 22-year-old single Hispanic woman who engages in nonsuicidal self-injury to manage feelings of anger, anxiety, and guilt. When she is angry at her boyfriend or another significant person in her life, she feels guilty for feeling angry; this leads to feelings of deep self-hatred, which she believes she cannot tolerate, and she begins to pinch her skin in order to feel physical pain that will distract her from these feelings. Sometimes the pinching leads to intense scratching until she draws blood. This provides a sense of relief from her emotions. The relief is experienced as feeling "back in control." CB describes two low-lethality suicide attempts that she distinguishes from the nonsuicidal self-injury. On two separate occasions, on the anniversary of the death of her father, she became extremely angry at her boyfriend for not acknowledging the difficulty of the day for her. She became hopeless, feeling that her boyfriend would never be able to understand her and that she would always feel unbearably sad about losing her father and would be unable to get the help she needed to deal with it. She also felt that there was something wrong with her for feeling this way. These thoughts led to a decision to take an overdose of her medication in order to kill herself. On both occasions, as soon as she took about 10 pills (not enough to cause lethal harm), she felt a sense of relief that at least she had done something to take control of her situation, and she no longer wished to die. She then fell asleep and had no other medical consequences from the overdose, and she woke up feeling much better.

Case Example 2

RJ is a 35-year-old single Caucasian woman who has made approximately 20 suicide attempts since she was 13 years old. At least 15 of these attempts have required medical attention and hospitalizations. RJ describes these attempts, as well as her chronic *suicidal ideation,* as her method of managing overwhelming feelings and avoiding confrontations and responsibility that she finds aversive. Many of the attempts occur without accompanying symptoms of depression. RJ's last attempt occurred during a period of self-reported *euthymic* mood and stability. RJ reports that she was in a good mood but became angry with her boyfriend over a few separate matters. Because RJ has difficulty being direct interpersonally and has problems experiencing or expressing her feelings, she avoided a confrontation with her boyfriend. However, she began to ruminate about the boyfriend's behavior and thereby continued to feed the very emotions that she was trying to avoid. RJ states that the feelings of anger became overwhelming and soon turned to fear and anxiety. RJ reports that, without much thought, she began taking prescription psychiatric medications one after another in a frantic effort to escape her state of misery. After taking a substantial number of pills, RJ reports that she realized she "blew it" and called her boss, a friend, and her therapist, hinting that she was in trouble. She then passed out. Soon emergency help arrived and took her to the hospital, where she needed medical care. After this attempt, as well as others, RJ appears bright, focused, and less anxious. She reports feeling motivated for change and willing to set goals, and she functions at an improved level. In addition, RJ reports that she feels regret for her actions because she recognizes that they disturb those whom she loves. These feelings, she reports, replace the anger she had felt previously. Likewise, RJ's loved ones seem interested, careful, and cognizant of her feelings. RJ reports that she feels more intimate with others and less fearful and alone. For a brief period lasting up to a month, RJ's emotional life feels manageable and enjoyable.

Discussion of Case Illustrations

It is clear that the conventional model of suicidality, as seen in major depression, does not apply to the suicidal behavior of the two individuals presented in these cases. In attempting to apply this model, clinicians may overlook the emotion-regulation function of suicidal behavior in these individuals. As stated earlier, this may lead to the erroneous conclusion that because the individual with BPD feels better afterward, the attempt was not as genuine or was intended purely to manipulate a caregiving response from others. This conclusion is especially likely to be drawn if the suicide attempt results in a markedly improved mood. It may be necessary to develop a different model for suicidal behavior in BPD so that risk and management can be accurately assessed.

The Self-Regulation Model of Self-Injury and Suicidal Behavior in BPD

Why do persons with BPD become suicidal, make suicide attempts, and engage in nonsuicidal self-injury? To answer this question, it is important to understand the daily experience of "being borderline." Individuals with BPD experience a pervasive sense of badness that can overwhelm them and that requires constant effort to resist. They feel buffeted about by their emotions; there is a sense of being controlled by, rather than being in control of, emotions. They also feel a deep sense of unworthiness and worthlessness that makes it difficult for them to tolerate disappointments and rejections. They have extreme difficulty "reading" and accepting inner states; they are very judgmental and demeaning of their reactions. They have a sense that their natural emotional reaction is incorrect, bad, stupid, wrong, terrible, and unnatural; this leads to self-invalidation and self-condemnation.

Zanarini et al. (1998) described the nature of the *dysphoria* experienced by individuals with BPD. Emotionally, compared with other individuals who have personality disorders, those with BPD spend a much higher percentage of time feeling overwhelmed, worthless, very angry, empty, abandoned, betrayed, furious, or enraged. Cognitively, individuals with BPD spend a higher percentage of time feeling misunderstood, thinking that no one cares or that they are bad, thinking about killing themselves, believing that they are evil, feeling like a small child, and believing they are damaged.

Leibenluft et al. (1987) mentioned several factors that predispose individuals with BPD to react to interpersonal stressors with self-injury. These authors suggested that the dysphoria experienced by these individuals has a primitive quality that belongs to an earlier developmental stage. Cognitive capabilities to recognize and verbally express dysphoric affect are absent or are not well developed, possibly as a result of early trauma that might have arrested cognitive development.

These experiences, feelings, and beliefs lead to a sense of badness that includes extreme self-criticism. These individuals maintain a very tenuous hold on their self-worth, which makes them particularly reliant on others for proof of their worthiness. Because their emotions are so dysregulated, they find upsets and disappointments very difficult to tolerate; and because of their reliance on others for worth, interpersonal difficulties are particularly upsetting to them. Therefore, pervasive feelings of badness and extreme self-criticism, along with tenuous self-worth bolstered by external forces, lead them to be extremely vulnerable to interpersonal disappointments, which are experienced as an assault on their tenuous self-esteem. They respond frantically, experiencing dysregulated anger both at the cause of upset and at themselves. These feelings of badness, anger at self, and self-criticism for being so vulnerable lead to suicidality and self-injury.

The self-regulation model proposes that self-injury and suicidal behavior serve a dual function in BPD: 1) to inflict physical harm; and 2) to regulate the self, particularly emotions, and to restore a sense of equilibrium and well-being. In this model, the individual experiences a range of unbearable emotions, thoughts, and feelings that are experienced as out of control and dysregulated. Self-condemnation for feeling so out of control frequently accompanies this state. This is a state of extreme misery that feels never-ending, even though it may last only a few hours. In response to this state, individuals feel they must do something to alter how they are feeling. The urge to act intensifies and is perceived as a reasonable solution. The result can be a suicide attempt or a self-injury episode. After the episode, individuals usually feel much more in control and often regain their sense of emotional equilibrium. Thus, the act is "successful" in that the regulation function has been fulfilled. This may explain why individuals with BPD feel better after self-injury episodes and suicide attempts. It also explains why hospitalization after an episode may not serve a helpful function.

● ● ●

In deciding whether or not to hospitalize, clinicians must perform a balancing act between taking the risk of suicide seriously and increasing patients' capacity to safely tolerate chronic suicidal ideation on their own.

● ● ●

Our new treatment model is based on an increased understanding of the phenomenology of BPD and self-injurious behavior in BPD. This improved understanding is necessary to treat and manage self-injury more effectively in this population. Improved treatment would address two areas of clinical work: 1) the reduction of self-injurious behavior and 2) risk assessment, including improving the ability to make decisions regarding hospitalization.

Reducing Self-Injurious Behavior

Our model could be applied in helping to reduce self-injury by informing a comprehensive assessment of the patient's subjective experience of self-injury with both suicidal and nonsuicidal intent. The following aspects of parasuicidal behavior would be evaluated:

1. **Function of the self-injury.** Rather than assuming that the intent and function of nonsuicidal self-injury is purely manipulative and attention seeking, a subjective assessment would allow for a more nuanced understanding of the various previously mentioned functions of both suicidal and nonsuicidal self-injury, such as emotion regulation, self-punishment, and self-validation. With the enhanced awareness of the multiple functions of parasuicidal behavior, treatment could focus on the development of more skillful ways to achieve these goals.

2. **Intent of past parasuicidal behaviors.** Assessment of intent associated with past parasuicidal behavior would include distinguishing between self-injurious acts performed with and without intent to die. Intent would not be inferred solely from the circumstances, the extent of medical lethality, or interpersonal consequences of the self-injurious event. Both the patient and the clinician would be encouraged to validate the individual's subjective report of his or her intent, despite objective circumstances that might seemingly contradict it.

3. **Cognitions and cognitive processes that contribute to self-injury.** As reviewed above (see "Cognitions and Cognitive Factors"), patients often have fixed or distorted beliefs that can lead to self-injury. For example, they may harbor the belief that they cannot tolerate emotional pain, or that the only way to handle their painful emotional state is through self-injury. Such beliefs, once recognized, can be modified through cognitive restructuring. Clinicians and patients can work together to understand how intense emotional arousal leads to distorted cognitions or interpretations of external events. Relatedly, therapeutic interventions can target increased awareness of how past traumatic events can distort the perceptions of current reality.

4. **Consequences of the self-injury.** Identifying the reinforcing consequences of the behavior can help the clinician understand the perpetuation of self-injury and can provide information about the ways to modify these reinforcement patterns to promote more skillful behaviors. In addition, distinguishing between intended and unintended consequences can aid both patient and clinician in clarifying original intent versus learned intent. Patients can gain more insight into how their behaviors affect the people close to them, which can provide an opportunity for improved interpersonal effectiveness.

Cognitive-behavioral treatments known to be effective in reducing self-injury in BPD, such as dialectical behavior therapy (DBT) and cognitive-behavioral therapy (CBT) (Beck 1995; Beck et al. 1979), incorporate many of these principles. Both DBT and CBT work to identify and correct distorted cognitions that lead to both the urge to self-injure and the propensity to act. DBT emphasizes the recognition of the reinforcing consequences that perpetuate maladaptive behaviors. DBT also targets emotion regulation (a common function of self-injury) and the decrease of self-criticism through validation and nonjudgmental thinking. In both DBT and CBT adapted for BPD, comprehensive analysis of the subjective experience of self-injury episodes is incorporated as a therapeutic intervention.

Risk Assessment and the Decision to Hospitalize

In deciding whether or not to hospitalize, clinicians must perform a balancing act between taking the risk of suicide seriously and increasing patients' capacity to safely tolerate, on their own, what is often chronic suicidal ideation. Here again, a more comprehensive assessment of the subjective experience of a self-injurious patient can aid in the difficult task of recognizing when the risk for suicide requires hospitalization.

As mentioned earlier, the chronic suicidal ideation and nonsuicidal self-injuring behavior prevalent among these patients, along with the tendency of clinicians and loved ones to experience the self-injury as attention seeking (whether intended or not), can result in reduced sensitivity to risk. Distinguishing between suicidal and nonsuicidal self-injury, which patients are often clearly able to do, can make both clinicians and patients better able to recognize actual suicide risk. In addition, recognizing the various functions of self-injury, not assuming the intent to be solely interpersonal, and maintaining awareness of the day-to-day emotional pain experienced by individuals with BPD can reduce the burnout that might lead to underrecognition of suicide risk.

On the other hand, chronic suicidal ideation and nonsuicidal self-injury also can lead to multiple hospitalizations that severely disrupt the individual's ability to function and that might be avoidable. We have stated that often, suicidal ideation and self-injurious behavior in BPD stem not necessarily from a strong intent to die, but rather from a desperate desire to manage and obtain relief from what feels like an intolerable emotional state. In other words, it can be an effort to stay alive. An outpatient treatment that can address the need for such relief and provide support for the individual to manage these states safely can reduce the need for revolving-door hospital admissions.

Gunderson and Ridolfi (2001) described a scenario in which multiple unnecessary hospitalizations result in a patient who comes to view hospitalization as the only way her pain can be validated and who presents herself as needing hospitalization even when the clinician does not believe it is necessary. Gunderson and Ridolfi present a principle of "false submission": the clinician agrees to hospitalize but works toward changing the meaning the patient ascribes to hospitalization. However, if hospitalization is to be used, it seems that the best time to hospitalize is for the very brief period when the individual is experiencing extreme distress that would normally lead up to a suicide attempt. In this instance, hospitalization would block the behavior and help the individual to tolerate the emotions until they subside.

Further Research

The self-regulation model we propose is distinct from existing models for major depression and other diagnostic groups. It is a model based on a comprehensive understanding of the subjective emotional, cognitive, and physiological experience of suicidal and nonsuicidal self-injury. Areas of further research that would contribute to the development and testing of the validity of this model include empirical studies of the differences in suicide attempts between individuals with BPD and those with major depression. In particular, suicidal intent among those with BPD and depressed suicide attempters should be assessed and compared. We might expect more ambivalence among attempters who have BPD, as well as more variation in intent from one attempt to another. Other variables to be compared would include reasons for making the attempt, level of medical lethality, number of lifetime attempts, level of depressed mood at the time of the attempt, identified environmental triggers leading to the attempt, and age at first suicide attempt.

Further studies documenting the phenomenology of self-mutilation are needed. In particular, research is needed to provide greater understanding of the role of neurocognitive processes and neurobiology in self-injury. This would include examining how distorted beliefs lead to self-injury and how emotional arousal affects cognition with regard to self-injury. Other areas where investigation is needed include those that could lead to a better understanding of the experience of pain and relief from pain, both emotional and physiological, in individuals with BPD.

What Families Need to Know

Key Messages in This Chapter

- Many individuals with BPD engage in nonsuicidal self-injuring behaviors (self-harm), have suicidal thoughts, and make suicide threats. This makes it very difficult for their family members and therapists to predict the actual risk for suicide.
- It is important not to overreact by believing that *every* act of self-injury (superficial cutting or burning of the skin, head banging, hair pulling, or skin picking) has suicidal intent. Suicide attempts and nonsuicidal self-injury are usually quite different in the mind of the person with BPD.
- It is equally important not to *underestimate* the risk of suicide in individuals with BPD. Self-mutilation (cutting or burning the skin) is itself

a risk factor for suicide: 55%–85% of self-mutilators have made at least one suicide attempt.

- The risk for completed suicide among individuals with BPD over their lifetimes is about 9%–10%.
- Rather than using self-injury to manipulate others and seek attention, many individuals with BPD are ashamed of the behavior and hide it from others.
- The trigger leading to self-injury in BPD is most often a real or perceived loss of a personal relationship through separation or abandonment.
- Among its possible functions, self-injury may actually help the person with BPD reduce emotional tension, distract him or her from feeling emotional pain, make the emotional suffering concrete and visible, or act on angry feelings. In other words, self-injury seems to help regulate emotions that are out of control.
- Many individuals with BPD who self-injure report an immediate sense of relief from emotional pressure afterward.
- The self-regulation model proposes that suicidal behavior and self-injury serve a dual function in BPD: to inflict physical harm *and* to regulate the emotions.
- During periods of extreme stress that could lead to a suicide attempt or self-injury episode, a stay in the hospital might block the behavior and help the person with BPD tolerate the emotions until they subside.

Key Words in This Chapter

affective   pertaining to one's emotional state.
affect regulation   controlling one's emotions.
analgesia   relief of pain.
clinical   concerned with the observation and treatment of disease.
cognition   a thought or belief.
depersonalization   a sense of being unreal.
dissociation   feelings of detachment from one's own body or thinking.
dysphoria   a state of sadness or depressed mood.
dysregulation   the inability to regulate or control (mood or impulses).
empirical   based on evidence, data, or experience.
endogenous opioids   substances found within the body that help control pain; for example, the endorphins.
euthymic   experiencing a normal or stable mood.
executive functioning   the ability to organize one's thoughts and reasoning skills.

ideation   the process of thinking or forming ideas.

neuroendocrine systems   hormone regulation in the brain; some psychiatric disorders are associated with the overactivity or underactivity of these hormones.

parasuicide   any self-injurious behavior, with or without suicidal intent, that does not result in death.

pathology   the condition and processes of a disease or disorder.

phenomenology   the observable features, in this case, of borderline personality disorder.

self-invalidation   the process of discounting or ignoring one's true feelings.

serotonin   a neurotransmitter (brain chemical) that can regulate affective symptoms (mood) and impulsive behavior.

suicidal ideation   thoughts of wishing one were not alive or of committing suicide.

References

Beck AT, Rush AJ, Shaw BF, et al: Cognitive Therapy of Depression. New York, Guilford, 1979

Beck JS: Cognitive Therapy: Basic and Beyond. New York, Guilford, 1995

Brodsky BS, Cloitre M, Dulit RA: Relationship of dissociation and childhood abuse in borderline personality disorder. Am J Psychiatry 152:1788–1792, 1995

Denning DG, Conwell Y, King D, et al: Method choice, intent, and gender in completed suicide. Suicide Life Threat Behav 30:282–288, 2000

Favazza AR: Why patients mutilate themselves. Hosp Community Psychiatry 40:137–140, 1989

Favazza AR, Conterio K: Female habitual self-mutilators. Acta Psychiatr Scand 79:283–289, 1989

Fine MA, Sansone RA: Dilemmas in the management of suicidal behavior in individuals with borderline personality disorder. Am J Psychother 44:160–171, 1990

Fyer M: Suicide attempts in patients with borderline personality disorder. Am J Psychiatry 145:737–739, 1988

Gardner AR, Gardner AJ: Self-mutilation, obsessionality and narcissism. Br J Psychiatry 127:127–132, 1975

Gardner DL, Cowdry RW: Suicidal and parasuicidal behavior in borderline personality disorder. Psychiatr Clin North Am 8:389–403, 1985

Gunderson JG: Borderline Personality Disorder. Washington, DC, American Psychiatric Press, 1984

Gunderson JG, Ridolfi M: Borderline personality disorder: suicidality and self-mutilation. Ann N Y Acad Sci 932:61–77, 2001

Keilp JG, Sackeim HA, Brodsky BS, et al: Neuropsychological dysfunction in depressed suicide attempters. Am J Psychiatry 158:735–741, 2001

Kemperman I, Russ MJ, Clark WC, et al: Pain assessment in self-injurious patients with borderline personality disorder using signal detection theory. Psychiatry Res 70:175–183, 1997

Leibenluft E, Gardner DL, Cowdry RW: The inner experience of the borderline self-mutilator. J Personal Disord 1:317–324, 1987

Linehan M: Cognitive-Behavioral Treatment of Borderline Personality Disorder. New York, Guilford, 1993

Linehan MM, Armstrong HE, Suarez A, et al: Cognitive-behavioral treatment of chronically parasuicidal borderline patients. Arch Gen Psychiatry 48:1060–1064, 1991

Rosenthal RJ, Rinzler C, Wallsh R, et al: Wrist-cutting syndrome: the meaning of a gesture. Am J Psychiatry 128:1363–1368, 1972

Roy A: Self-mutilation. Br J Med Psychol 51:201–203, 1978

Russ MJ: Self-injurious behavior in patients with borderline personality disorder: biological perspectives. J Personal Disord 6:64–81, 1992

Russ MJ, Shearin EN, Clarkin JF, et al: Subtypes of self-injurious patients with borderline personality disorder. Am J Psychiatry 150:1869–1871, 1993

Sachsse U, Von der Heyde S, Huether G: Stress regulation and self-mutilation (case report). Am J Psychiatry 159:672, 2002

Shearer SL: Phenomenology of self-injury among inpatient women with borderline personality disorder. J Nerv Ment Dis 182:524–526, 1994

Shearer SL, Peter CP, Quaytman MS, et al: Intent and lethality of suicide attempts among female borderline inpatients. Am J Psychiatry 145:1424–1427, 1988

Soloff PH, Lis JA, Kelly T, et al: Self-mutilation and suicidal behavior in borderline personality disorder. J Personal Disord 8:257–267, 1994

Stanley B, Gameroff MJ, Michalsen V, et al: Are suicide attempters who self-mutilate a unique population? Am J Psychiatry 158:427–432, 2001

Stanley B, Sher L, Ekman R, et al: Self-injurious behavior and endogenous opioid levels in cerebrospinal fluid. Paper presented at the International Association of Suicide Prevention, Stockholm, Sweden, September 2003

Stone MH, Hurt SW, Stone DK: The PI 500: long-term follow-up of borderline inpatients meeting DSM-III criteria, I: global outcome. J Personal Disord 1:291–298, 1987a

Stone MH, Stone DK, Hurt SW: Natural history of borderline patients treated by intensive hospitalization. Psychiatr Clin North Am 10:185–206, 1987b

Suyemoto KL: The functions of self-mutilation. Clin Psychol Rev 18:531–554, 1998

Ventura SJ, Peters KD, Martin JA, et al: Births and deaths: United States, 1996. Mon Vital Stat Rep 46 (1 suppl 2):1–40, 1997

Winchel R, Stanley M: Self-injurious behavior: a review of the behavior and biology of self-mutilation. Am J Psychiatry 148:306–317, 1991

Zanarini MC, Frankenburg FR, DeLuca CJ, et al: The pain of being borderline: dysphoric states specific to borderline personality disorder. Harv Rev Psychiatry 6:201–207, 1998

• 4 •

Pharmacotherapy in Borderline Personality Disorder

Paul H. Soloff, M.D.

Personality disorders are best viewed as complex *syndromes* resulting from the interaction of biological and learned influences on perception, cognition, affect, and behavior. By convention, personality dimensions associated with learned behavior are referred to as traits of *character.* These are attitudes, values, moral beliefs, and expectations derived from cultural, social, familial, and interpersonal experiences. Dimensions of personality believed to have a more direct biological *etiology,* whether inherited or acquired, are generally referred to as traits of *temperament.*

Although it is customary to discuss personality dimensions in contradictory terms—such as "temperament versus character," "learned versus inherited," or "nature versus nurture"—it is important to recognize that all dimensions of personality are closely interrelated throughout development. For example, a child born with an impulsive or aggressive temperament will interact with the world differently than one born with an avoidant or shy temperament and will develop attitudes, expectations, and interpersonal behaviors conditioned by this experience. Similarly, the attitudes, values, and expectations of the family expressed in their child-rearing practices will shape the behavioral expression of temperamental *impulsivity* and aggressivity.

• • •

A child born with an impulsive or aggressive temperament will interact with the world differently than one born with an avoidant or shy temperament and will develop attitudes, expectations, and interpersonal behaviors conditioned by this experience.

• • •

Although painful life events such as trauma or loss can be considered learned experience, they may also have a **pathogenic** effect on brain development early in life, and hence on temperament. For example, children who experience severe maltreatment early in life undergo changes in the function of the neuroendocrine system of the brain that persist into adulthood. Regulatory responses of this neuroendocrine system (the hypothalamic-pituitary-adrenal system) are persistently altered. These children also have persisting decreases in the size of the hippocampus, an important brain structure that is involved in memory (De Bellis et al. 1999a, 1999b; Stein et al. 1997). Adult women with borderline personality disorder (BPD) who have had childhood experiences of maltreatment, especially sexual abuse, have reduction in the volume of the hippocampus and the amygdala, as well as diminished responsiveness of *serotonin* function (Driessen et al. 2000; Rinne et al. 2000). The amygdala is important in regulation of affect, especially anger, whereas the serotonin system is involved in the regulation and inhibition of affect, impulse, and behavior. These acquired abnormalities in neuroendocrine and neurotransmitter regulation and in brain structure and function ultimately have significant effects on behavior.

Role of Neurotransmitters in Brain Function

Temperamental traits such as impulsivity or affective instability are regulated by chemical signals in the brain, conducted by substances called *neurotransmitters.* Neurotransmitters regulate many basic brain functions, affecting the ways people perceive and think about the world, experience and express emotion, and regulate their actions. The regulation of mood and behavior depends on a chemical balance in specific neural circuits in the brain. Temperamental traits such as impulsivity and affective instability may be expressed in maladaptive ways because of inborn or acquired imbalances in the neural circuits that regulate their expression. The neurotransmitter chemistry of these neural circuits and the modulation of some temperamental traits appear to be responsive to pharmacological manipulation. In individuals with BPD, poorly regulated expressions of these temperamental traits (e.g., impulsive aggression, affective instability, suicidal and *parasuicidal* behavior) are easily recognized as target symptoms of treatment.

● ● ●

Because BPD is a syndrome, not a disease, multiple medications are sometimes necessary to target symptoms that arise from different chemistries.

● ● ●

BPD is a syndrome defined by a cluster of personality traits and associated behaviors. It is not a disease in the medical sense, with a single biological cause. Among the defining characteristics, impulsivity and affective dysregulation appear to be the core biological components. Mild distortions of thinking and perception also may be present and may have a basis in neurotransmitter function. Because BPD is a syndrome, a pharmacological approach to its treatment must be symptom specific. Medications are targeted against the neurotransmitter basis of affective, impulsive, or *cognitive* symptoms and the biology that gives rise to such symptoms at times of stress.

Some Basic Principles in the Pharmacotherapy of BPD

The symptom domains that constitute the targets for *pharmacotherapy* in BPD may be broken into three large categories: 1) cognitive-perceptual symptoms, 2) affective dysregulation, and 3) impulsive behavioral symptoms. Each of these large symptom domains appears to be mediated, in part, by neurotransmitter functions that are amenable to pharmacological manipulation.

Because BPD is a syndrome, not a disease, multiple medications are sometimes necessary to target symptoms that arise from different chemistries. However, many medications have a broad range of effects and treat multiple symptoms. For example, the *selective serotonin reuptake inhibitor (SSRI) antidepressants* help with both impulsive aggression and depression. The best practice is to introduce one medication at a time and see the full scope of effects before adding a second or third drug. The addition of too many medications too quickly may make it difficult to distinguish which one is helping and increase the risk of drug interactions and side effects. Medications that are not helpful should be discontinued rather than being allowed to accumulate in the body.

Pharmacotherapy in BPD is **adjunctive** to a comprehensive multidimensional psychosocial approach to the treatment of the person. It is important to note that pharmacotherapy does not target the disturbed and unstable interpersonal relationships of the individual with BPD, which are the proper dominion of psychotherapy. However, many patients (and their therapists) find that the relief of cognitive, **affective**, and impulsive symptoms through the judicious use of medication makes it possible for them to engage more effectively in psychotherapy.

Limitations of Treatment Studies

To better understand treatment recommendations, it is important to understand the problems and limitations in conducting pharmacotherapy studies in BPD. Patients with BPD who are admitted to research trials from which our treatment recommendations are derived may not be typical of the average person with BPD. BPD often coexists with affective disorders such as major depression, dysthymic disorder, and (less commonly) bipolar disorder. Patients with other coexisting disorders may be excluded from research trials. If they are included, it is often difficult for the clinician to differentiate the chronic mood symptoms and low self-esteem belonging to the BPD syndrome from similar symptoms belonging to the superimposed illness.

The type of reimbursement for care can also place limitations on treatment studies. In many areas, treatment reimbursed under managed care insurance must be split into component parts, each separately reimbursed. Psychotherapy is conducted by psychologists, social workers, and credentialed therapists, whereas medical diagnoses and pharmacological management are provided by psychiatrists. BPD patients may attend dialectical behavior therapy groups and see therapists and psychiatrists in separate settings.

One consequence of this arrangement is that the psychiatrist usually sees the patient less frequently and for shorter periods of time than the therapist. Judgments about medication **efficacy** based solely on the patient's account may be inaccurate. In some research studies, patients report little subjective change, whereas professionals see significant improvements in behavior. It is important that the psychiatrist be kept abreast of critical changes in the patient's symptom patterns and behavior between medical assessments. An agreement with the patient to allow contact between professionals is critical to effective care in any split-care arrangement and must be negotiated as part of the therapeutic contract at the beginning of treatment.

● ● ●

Medication does not change character and should be viewed as part of a comprehensive treatment plan, which may include psychotherapy and psychoeducation.

● ● ●

Pharmacotherapies and Their Use in BPD

The recommendations for pharmacotherapy in BPD presented in this chapter are derived from review of the existing *empirical* literature, consensus among members of the American Psychiatric Association (2001) practice guideline work group and its reviewers, and my own years of experience in studying BPD. It is important to recognize that recommendations for pharmacological management are based on a relatively small number of studies. The American Psychiatric Association work group that wrote the *Practice Guideline for the Treatment of Patients with Borderline Personality Disorder* found only 40–50 published scientific reports on the drug treatment of BPD. This is a woefully inadequate database. Through this experience it has been learned that drug effects in BPD are modest and that residual symptoms are the rule. *Medication does not change character and should be viewed as an adjunctive part of a comprehensive psychosocial treatment plan, which may include psychotherapy and psychoeducation.* This section describes the medications used to treat each of the three symptom domains in BPD: cognitive symptoms, affective dysregulation, and impulsivity.

Cognitive-Perceptual Symptoms

The cognitive-perceptual symptoms of BPD are most commonly expressed at times of severe emotional stress. These symptoms include undue suspiciousness; *ideas of reference* and paranoid ideas; and transient distortions in perception, such as illusions and brief auditory or visual hallucinations. Some individuals with BPD have out-of-body experiences—that is, seeing oneself from a distance (depersonalization)—or feelings that the world around them has become unreal, as though it is being viewed through a fog or a window (derealization). Some patients have more chronic distortions in thinking, including beliefs that appear odd or eccentric (e.g., beliefs in a "sixth sense" or magical abilities). The neurotransmitter *dopamine* has been implicated in the expression of some of the psychotic-like symptoms or the so-called mild thought disorders seen in BPD. Dopamine may also be involved in the mediation of arousal, irritability, and anger. Dopamine-blocking medications, the *neuroleptics,* are the treatment of first choice for these symptoms.

Neuroleptic Medications

In the person with BPD, neuroleptic medications have been shown to have a very broad spectrum of effects, reducing symptom severity in all three symptom domains. However, they have their greatest effect and are most specific for cognitive and perceptual symptoms. Neuroleptic medications are also highly effective against the anger, irritability, and hostility that often accompany these cognitive-perceptual symptoms.

● ● ●

In the person with BPD, neuroleptic medications have been shown to have a very broad spectrum of effects, reducing symptom severity in all three symptom domains.

● ● ●

There is more scientific evidence for the efficacy of neuroleptic medications in the treatment of BPD symptoms than for any other drug class. In general, the relevant research studies have used low doses of neuroleptic drugs for study periods of 5–24 weeks. One exceptionally long study, using an injectable form of antipsychotic medication, lasted 6 months and demonstrated favorable effects against recurrent suicidality in patients with histrionic and borderline personality disorders (Montgomery and Montgomery 1982). Because the onset of action for neuroleptic drugs is typically rapid—hours to days depending on the method of administration—the psychiatrist may recommend neuroleptics for short-term use during times of crisis. For example, an effect against anger and aggression may be obtained within hours, especially with intramuscular use.

Side effects.   Many of the older antipsychotic medications are associated with unpleasant side effects, even at low doses. Side effects of these medications commonly include muscle stiffness and a slowed, shuffling gait, as in Parkinson's disease; muscle restlessness and tremor (**akathisia**), which could easily be mistaken for anxiety; and, less commonly, involuntary muscle spasms (dystonic reactions), especially of the neck and eye muscles. These effects are associated more frequently with high-potency drugs such as haloperidol (Haldol) and thiothixene (Navane), two drugs that have been studied in patients with BPD. Low-potency **antipsychotics,** such as chlorpromazine (Thorazine), and thioridazine (Mellaril) also have been used in research studies in BPD and are associated with sedation, dry mouth, constipation, and postural hypotension (a sudden decrease in blood pressure on standing).

Atypical Neuroleptics

It is important for families to appreciate that side effects are often responsible for noncompliance with drug treatments. Fortunately, the more recent additions to the antipsychotic pharmacy, called *atypical* neuroleptics, have minimal side effects and are very well tolerated in low doses. Olanzapine (Zyprexa) and risperidone (Risperdal) have been studied in patients with BPD in doses of 2.5–10 mg/day for olanzapine and 2.5–4.0 mg/day for risperidone. Olanzapine is often associated with weight gain (if food intake is not monitored carefully) and is mildly sedating, whereas risperidone in higher doses (i.e., greater than 6 mg) can cause muscle symptoms similar to those caused by older neuroleptics.

One atypical antipsychotic medication deserves special consideration. Clozapine (Clozaril) was the first atypical antipsychotic to be developed and is arguably the most potent of this class of drugs. Clozapine has been shown to reverse serious symptoms of disordered thinking and perception after other antipsychotic medications have failed. Although it is used most widely in the treatment of **refractory** schizophrenia, clozapine has also been used successfully in the treatment of patients with BPD whose cognitive-perceptual symptoms or impulsive behavioral symptoms (including impulsive self-mutilation) have not responded to conventional antipsychotic medications (Frankenburg and Zanarini 1993). In rare cases, clozapine is associated with suppression of the white blood cell count to dangerously low levels. Because this is a potentially life-threatening side effect, all patients taking clozapine must be enrolled in a special program that monitors white blood cell counts. For this reason, clozapine is often considered a treatment of last resort.

Side effects. Long-term use of older neuroleptics is associated with development of a persistent neurological movement disorder called *tardive dyskinesia,* which is characterized by slow, rhythmic, automatic movements. At present the newer atypical medications are not thought to cause tardive dyskinesia. Research indicates that even low-dose neuroleptics may be poorly tolerated over extended periods of time. Once the acute symptoms are in remission, the patient may become progressively intolerant of side effects and may discontinue follow-up. In general, neuroleptic medication should be used briefly, usually weeks to months, to produce remission of target symptoms. Some clinicians use low-dose neuroleptics as an adjunct to anger management on a long-term basis (the patient's "anger pill"). There are currently no published studies of the maintenance use of neuroleptic medications in BPD. Long-term use is a matter of clinical judgment.

Symptoms of Affective Dysregulation

Affective *dysregulation* is expressed as marked reactivity or *lability* of mood and can involve angry, depressive, or anxious feelings. The intense and inappropriate anger of the person with BPD is so characteristic that it is included as a diagnostic criterion for the disorder. In its extreme form, this anger can be expressed in temper tantrums, physical assaults, destruction of property, or self-injury. The suicidal behavior of borderline patients is often motivated more by anger than by depression (Soloff et al. 1994). The sensitivity to rejection and depressive "mood crashes" also result from an inability to regulate mood, which may be related to decreased regulation of the neurotransmitter serotonin in the brain. Medications that increase serotonin transmission, such as the SSRIs, elevate its level in the brain and help to modulate some of these symptoms.

SSRI Antidepressants

SSRI antidepressants are the treatment of first choice for affective dysregulation involving depressive moods, anger, and anxiety. They also have a distinct effect against impulsive aggression and, in some cases, self-injurious behavior. In some studies of SSRI antidepressants, modest improvement across all three symptom domains has been demonstrated. Evidence for the efficacy of SSRIs and related antidepressants comes from studies conducted with both inpatients and outpatients using medications such as fluoxetine (Prozac), sertraline (Zoloft), and venlafaxine (Effexor). These medications are commonly given in the same doses required for treating depression and have been tested in research trials lasting anywhere from 6 to 14 weeks. The time of response—several weeks—is similar to that seen in the treatment of depression. Several research trials have noted that the effects of the SSRI antidepressants on dysregulated mood are separate from the effects on impulsive aggression. Effects on impulsive aggression appear much earlier than effects on depressed mood. Similarly, when the drugs are discontinued, impulsive aggression can reappear within days.

● ● ●

SSRI antidepressants are the treatment of first choice for affective dysregulation involving depressive moods, anger, and anxiety.

● ● ●

Side effects. The advent of the SSRI antidepressants marked a major advance in the care of depressed and anxious patients. Because of the lack of major side effects, these medications (Prozac, Zoloft, Paxil, Celexa, and others) were much easier to tolerate than the older generation of medications (e.g., the tricyclic antidepressants) and found rapid acceptance among physicians and patients. These drugs are also much less dangerous in overdose. Although side effects can vary in degree from drug to drug, those common to the class of SSRI medications can include mild, transient nausea; dry mouth; constipation or diarrhea; insomnia or somnolence; loss of appetite; restlessness (akathisia); tremor; and increased sweating. With very widespread use of these medications, physicians have become aware of a less common but disturbing side effect that can lead to noncompliance: the inhibition of sexual drive or performance. It is important to recognize that restlessness (akathisia) can be caused by SSRI medications, as noted above. This restlessness should not be ignored or misdiagnosed as increased anxiety, because it has been associated with suicidal behavior.

If an SSRI medication does not produce the desired result in 4–6 weeks, a second trial of a different SSRI medication is recommended. Given the favorable side-effect profile of the SSRIs, this so-called salvage strategy is widely used in the treatment of depressed mood. Research has indicated that patients may be sensitive to a second SSRI medication even after a first trial in which they did not respond.

Monoamine Oxidase Inhibitor Antidepressants

The *monoamine oxidase inhibitor (MAOI) antidepressants* are an older family of antidepressant medications that are more difficult to use than the SSRIs. MAOI antidepressants have demonstrated efficacy against affective dysregulation in BPD in a similar number of controlled drug trials to the SSRI antidepressants. However, because of dangers inherent in their use,

MAOI antidepressants are not recommended as first-line treatments for affective dysregulation in BPD. Patients taking MAOI antidepressants must carefully follow a diet low in tyramine, because tyramine causes elevated blood pressure if too much is absorbed. (The MAOI antidepressants interfere with the normal metabolism of tyramine and chemically related substances.) Foods containing high levels of tyramine include aged cheeses, beer, red wine, liqueurs, hard salami and other dry fermented sausages, beef or chicken liver, fava beans, and smoked or pickled fishes (e.g., herring). Some common medications must be avoided, including most decongestants (e.g., pseudoephedrine, phenylephrine), meperidine (Demerol, a pain medication), and some older antihypertensive drugs (e.g., reserpine, methyldopa, guanethidine). Some street drugs are especially dangerous to patients taking MAOI antidepressants; these include cocaine and "speed" or "uppers" of the amphetamine family.

● ● ●

The doctor prescribing MAOI antidepressants should provide the patient with a list of the foods and medications to be avoided while taking these medications. It is essential that the family also be aware of these foods and medicines.

● ● ●

If taken in overdose, the MAOI antidepressants can be quite toxic. Although psychiatrists should consider an SSRI antidepressant as the first-line treatment for affective dysregulation, the MAOI antidepressants should be considered if the SSRI is ineffective. MAOI antidepressants are often quite helpful in cases of refractory depression, especially the atypical pattern seen most often in BPD. Used properly, they are very valuable therapeutic agents. Again, judgment is required, because the cooperation of patient and family are essential with this family of medicines.

Research trials studying the MAOIs have lasted from 5 to 16 weeks. The doctor prescribing MAOI antidepressants should provide the patient with a list of foods and medications to avoid while taking these medications. It is essential that family members also be aware of these foods and medicines. When buying over-the-counter medications, it is useful to ask the store pharmacist about possible drug interactions with MAOIs. The treating psychiatrist should also advise the patient as to the symptoms of hypertensive crisis and what steps to take should this occur. Treatment of elevated blood pressure may involve a simple remedy such as taking a rapid-acting antihypertensive medicine such as nifedipine (Procardia) or may involve a visit to the doctor or emergency room.

Side effects.   Phenelzine (Nardil) and tranylcypromine (Parnate) are the most commonly available MAOI antidepressants used in psychiatry. In general, tranylcypromine is a highly activating agent, whereas phenelzine is associated more often with sedation. Apart from the tyramine-food interaction, these antidepressants have some common side effects. For tranylcypromine, these include postural hypotension and fainting (at higher doses), overstimulation, restlessness, insomnia or drowsiness, and weakness. Side effects of phenelzine include postural hypotension, drowsiness, fatigue, tremors, headache, dry mouth, constipation, weight gain, disturbances in sexual performance, and *edema.* Newer MAOI medications are being introduced that minimize the risks of hypertensive crises, although these medications are not yet available in the United States.

● ● ●

Despite surprisingly little research support for their use, antianxiety medications are widely prescribed for borderline patients. These medications are subject to much abuse and can become addictive.

● ● ●

Antianxiety Medications

Although there is surprisingly little research support for their use, antianxiety medications are widely prescribed for BPD patients. Medications such as alprazolam (Xanax), lorazepam (Ativan), and clonazepam (Klonopin) are frequently used against the acute and chronic manifestations of anxiety in BPD. These medications, part of the *benzodiazepine* family, are subject to much abuse and can become addictive. Sudden discontinuation of these drugs after prolonged use can lead to withdrawal symptoms, including seizures. A randomized trial conducted at the National Institute of Mental Health found that Xanax, a benzodiazepine with a very short half-life, was associated with severe *disinhibition* and worsening of behavior in a majority of outpatient women with BPD who took the drug in a controlled manner (Gardner and Cowdry 1986). The disinhibited behavior, which included self-destructive acts and violence directed toward others, remains a significant clinical concern for the use of these medicines in BPD. Clonazepam, a benzodiazepine with a very long half-life, may be an exception to this pattern, perhaps as a result of its enhancement of serotonin neurotransmission. Clonazepam has been reported to be useful against agitation and aggression in case reports of severely ill patients.

At present there are no published research trials in borderline patients for the serotonergic antianxiety medication buspirone (Buspar), which does not cause chemical dependence. The benefits of buspirone are slow to develop, and weeks are often required for maximal efficacy. In my experience, this delay is often unacceptable to patients who want rapid relief.

Mood Stabilizers

Mood stabilizers, which are indicated primarily for the treatment of bipolar disorders, can also be useful in the treatment of affective instability in individuals with BPD. Because mood stabilizers are indicated for both affective dysregulation and impulsive behavior, they are described in detail below under "Impulsive Behavioral Symptoms."

Impulsive Behavioral Symptoms

Impulsive behavioral symptoms in BPD can include self-destructive behavior or impulsive aggression against oneself or others or against property. Impulsivity is a major risk factor for suicidal behavior, often in the context of anger, loss, or perceived rejection. Impulsivity may be expressed behaviorally in binges of spending, eating, drug use, or sexual activity. Some individuals with BPD are reckless drivers, accumulating speeding tickets and becoming involved in accidents. Impulsivity can also be reflected cognitively in rash judgments. Disinhibition of affect and impulse may have common elements in neurotransmitter chemistry (e.g., the neurotransmission of serotonin may be involved in the control of both impulse and affect). Treatments that are helpful for affective dysregulation may also help with behavioral symptoms.

SSRI Antidepressants

The SSRI antidepressants are the drugs of first choice for the treatment of impulsive behavioral symptoms in individuals with BPD. As in the treatment of affective dysregulation, failure of the SSRI antidepressants should prompt consideration of the MAOI antidepressants (which also can help with impulsive behavior), followed by consideration of the mood stabilizers. Many clinicians find that a combination of antidepressant medication and mood stabilizers is helpful in treating this important behavioral dimension. When rapid action is needed, as in the case of an angry, impulsive, and potentially violent patient, the short-term use of low-dose neuroleptics, even by intramuscular injection, may be required.

Mood Stabilizers

Several studies conducted with inpatients and outpatients in adult and adolescent populations have demonstrated utility for mood-stabilizing medications in the treatment of behavioral symptoms. These medications are given at usual clinical dose ranges and durations of 4–6 weeks for research trials. These medications—lithium carbonate, divalproex sodium (Depakote), and carbamazepine (Tegretol, Carbatrol)—have defined therapeutic blood levels derived from work with bipolar disorders.

● ● ●

Depakote, an anticonvulsant mood stabilizer widely used in treatment of bipolar disorder, has been shown to be useful against unstable mood and aggressive behavior in BPD.

● ● ●

Lithium has a very narrow therapeutic range, so too much medication can quickly cause significant side effects, and overdose can be fatal. In the normal therapeutic doses and blood range, common side effects may include initial nausea, thirst, a fine tremor, drowsiness, and muscle weakness. Long-term effects can include a reversible suppression of the thyroid gland, which must be monitored periodically through blood testing.

Carbamazepine is an anticonvulsant medication that is used for both mood dysregulation and behavioral symptoms in BPD. It has been used to treat impulsive aggression in patients with personality disorder, especially in the presence of an abnormal electroencephalogram (EEG). Periodic blood monitoring is needed to determine therapeutic plasma blood levels and possible adverse effects. Common side effects of carbamazepine include nausea, drowsiness, double or blurred vision, unsteady gait, headache, and fatigue. Side effects usually diminish over time. A recently introduced modification of this medication, oxcarbazepine (Trileptal), may be tolerated more easily.

Divalproex sodium (Depakote), an anticonvulsant mood stabilizer that is widely used in the treatment of bipolar disorder, has been shown to be useful against unstable mood and aggressive behavior in BPD (Hollander et al. 2001). As with other medications of this group, divalproex requires periodic blood-level monitoring and can be titrated against a therapeutic blood level. Research trials to determine its efficacy against impulsivity have typically lasted 6–10 weeks. Common side effects can include stomach upset, sedation, tremor, hair loss, and weight gain or loss.

Duration of Pharmacotherapy

How long does one continue medication in the treatment of BPD? The duration of research trials provides only a very rough outline for the minimum time to test the efficacy of any medication. Continuation and long-term maintenance of these medications have not been subjected to research study. For treatment of cognitive-perceptual symptoms with low-dose neuroleptics, a short-term strategy—that is, weeks to months—appears most realistic. For treatment of affective dysregulation and impulsive behavioral symptoms, the duration of treatment is more difficult to define. These are traits of the patient's temperament expressed as clinical symptoms because of a loss of conscious control. A useful strategy for the clinician is to keep the patient on a successful medication regimen until psychotherapy has fostered new coping strategies. In short, patients must stay under medication control until they learn to cope with the stresses that precipitated symptoms in the past.

Afterword

Note: The U.S. Food and Drug Administration has not approved BPD as an indication for any medication. All recommendations made in this chapter, although based on available evidence, are "off-label" recommendations. (Indications for the use of pharmacotherapy in BPD are summarized in Table 4–1.) All medication treatments used in BPD should be considered empirical treatment trials, with doctor and patient collaborating in the treatment effort and in the assessment of efficacy. Expectations for pharmacotherapy should be realistic. Pharmacotherapy does not treat disturbed interpersonal relations but may be a valuable adjunct to the work of psychotherapy in changing the character of the individual with BPD.

Table 4–1.   Indications for use of pharmacotherapy in borderline personality disorder

Symptom type	Symptom-specific pharmacotherapies
Cognitive-perceptual (psychotic-like) symptoms	
1. Suspiciousness, paranoid ideation, ideas of reference	**First choice:** low-dose neuroleptics, including new atypical agents (clozapine as treatment of last resort for psychotic-like symptoms)
2. Illusions, dissociation, stress-related hallucinations (and associated anger, hostility, irritability)	
Symptoms of affective dysregulation	
1. Reactive, depressed, anxious moods	**First choice:** selective serotonin reuptake inhibitors (SSRIs; e.g., fluoxetine, sertraline) and related antidepressants (e.g., venlafaxine)
2. Lability, affective instability, "mood crashes," rejection sensitivity, "mood swings"	**Second choice:** monoamine oxidase inhibitors (MAOIs; phenelzine, tranylcypromine)
3. Irritability, anger, hostility, temper outbursts	**Third choice:** mood stabilizers (lithium carbonate, divalproex sodium, carbamazepine (may be adjunctive or monotherapy)
	(Adjunctive use: neuroleptics for urgent control of anger, clonazepam for anxiety)
Symptoms of impulsive-behavioral dyscontrol	
1. Impulsive aggression	**First choice:** SSRIs and related antidepressants
2. Impulsive suicidal threats, gestures, self-injurious behaviors	(Adjunctive use: low-dose neuroleptics for anger, assaultiveness)
	Second choice: MAOIs *or* lithium carbonate
3. Impulsive binge behaviors (e.g., food, spending, drugs)	**Third choice:** divalproex sodium, carbamazepine (may be adjunctive to antidepressants or monotherapy)
	Fourth choice: clozapine

What Families Need to Know

Key Messages in This Chapter

- BPD is not a disease in the medical sense, with a single biological cause. Rather, it is a syndrome (a group of symptoms), so multiple medications may be needed to target these symptoms specifically.
- Temperamental traits such as impulsivity or instability of mood (affective instability)—some of the symptoms of BPD—are regulated by chemical signals in the brain, called neurotransmitters. Specific medications may target imbalances in these chemicals and thereby alleviate symptoms.
- Recommendations of specific medications to control BPD symptoms are based on a relatively small number of studies; drug effects are modest, and symptoms often return.
- Long-term use of these medications has not been studied. People with BPD may need to continue taking their medications until they learn to cope with the stresses that make their symptoms worse.
- Relief of cognitive, affective, and impulsive symptoms through pharmacotherapy often makes it possible for individuals with BPD to engage more successfully in psychotherapy as part of a comprehensive psychosocial treatment plan.

Key Words in This Chapter

adjunctive   added to or joined with other treatments.

affective   pertaining to one's emotional state.

akathisia   restlessness.

antipsychotics   medications that target symptoms of psychosis or thought disorders.

benzodiazepines   medications used to treat anxiety; they are often subject to abuse and can become addictive.

cognitive   pertaining to thinking.

disinhibition   a failure in the ability to control behaviors or feelings.

dopamine   a chemical in the brain that may be associated with the cognitive (disordered thinking) symptoms in BPD.

dysregulation   malfunction in the ability to regulate or control (often applied to mood or impulses).

edema   swelling of body tissues with fluids.

efficacy   effectiveness (of a treatment).

empirical   based on evidence or experience (in this chapter, with the use of medications).

etiology   cause or presumed cause.

ideas of reference   a disordered perception in which an individual falsely believes that others (or the television or radio) are speaking to or about him or her.

impulsivity   inability to resist performing some action.

lability   rapid fluctuation, instability, changeability.

monoamine oxidase inhibitor (MAOI) antidepressants   a class of anti-depressants shown to be effective in regulating affective (emotional) symptoms; certain foods and other medications are prohibited while taking these medications.

mood stabilizers   medications used mainly for bipolar disorder that can help regulate both affective symptoms and impulsive behaviors in BPD.

neuroleptics   antipsychotic medications that block the action of dopamine.

neurotransmitters   chemical signals in the brain that affect the way humans perceive the world, regulate their emotions, and control their actions.

parasuicidal   pertaining to any self-injurious behavior, with or without suicidal intent, that does not result in death.

pathogenic   causing disease.

pharmacotherapy   treatment with medications.

refractory   resistant to treatment.

selective serotonin reuptake inhibitor (SSRI) antidepressants   medications that increase the transmission of serotonin in the brain; they may both alleviate affective (mood) symptoms and help control impulsive behavior.

serotonin   a neurotransmitter or brain chemical that can regulate affective (mood) symptoms and impulsive behavior.

syndrome   a group of symptoms that together characterize a particular disorder.

References

American Psychiatric Association: Practice Guideline for the Treatment of Patients With Borderline Personality Disorder. Washington, DC, American Psychiatric Association, 2001

De Bellis MD, Baum AS, Birmaher B, et al: A.E. Bennett Research Award. Developmental traumatology, part I: biological stress systems. Biol Psychiatry 45:1259–1270, 1999a

De Bellis MD, Keshavan MS, Clark DB, et al: A.E. Bennett Research Award. Developmental traumatology, part II: brain development. Biol Psychiatry 45:1271–1284, 1999b

Driessen M, Herrmann J, Stahl K, et al: Magnetic resonance imaging volumes of the hippocampus and the amygdala in women with borderline personality disorder and early traumatization. Arch Gen Psychiatry 57:1115–1122, 2000

Frankenburg F, Zanarini M: Clozapine treatment of borderline patients: a preliminary study. Compr Psychiatry 34:402–405, 1993

Gardner DL, Cowdry RW: Development of melancholia during carbamazepine treatment in borderline personality disorder. J Clin Psychopharmacol 6:236–239, 1986

Hollander E, Allen A, Lopez RP, et al: A preliminary double-blind, placebo-controlled trial of divalproex sodium in borderline personality disorder. J Clin Psychiatry 62:199–203, 2001

Montgomery SA, Montgomery D: Pharmacologic prevention of suicidal behavior. J Affect Disord 4:291–298, 1982

Rinne T, Westenberg HG, den Boer JA, et al: Serotonergic blunting to *meta*-chlorophenylpiperazine (m-CPP) highly correlates with sustained childhood abuse in impulsive and autoaggressive female borderline patients. Biol Psychiatry 47:548–556, 2000

Soloff PH, Lis JA, Kelly T, et al: Risk factors for suicidal behavior in borderline personality disorder. Am J Psychiatry 151:1316–1323, 1994

Stein MB, Koverola C, Hanna C, et al: Hippocampal volume in women victimized by childhood sexual abuse. Psychol Med 27:951–959, 1997

• 5 •

The Longitudinal Course of Borderline Personality Disorder

Mary C. Zanarini, Ed.D.

Despite overwhelming evidence that borderline personality disorder (BPD) is a serious public health problem, little is known about its long-term symptomatic and psychosocial outcome. Even less is known about why some people with BPD make substantial progress, some hold their own, some deteriorate, and some commit suicide. Admittedly, the number of studies examining the *prognosis* for people with BPD is extremely small compared with the number of such studies that have been conducted in schizophrenia or bipolar disorder. To date, only 17 small-scale, short-term *prospective studies* and four large-scale, long-term *follow-back (retrospective) studies* of the course of BPD have been conducted. However, only large-scale, long-term prospective studies of the course of BPD will permit a naturalistic assessment of the outcome of the disorder as well as the factors most closely associated with improvement or lack of improvement. In the past decade, only two such methodologically rigorous studies have been undertaken. In this chapter I review the results of these three distinct groups of studies.

Small-Scale, Short-Term Prospective Studies of the Course of BPD

Early Studies: 1960s–1970s

Early studies of the course of BPD looked at the social functioning, employment status, and re-hospitalization of very small numbers (14–41) of people hospitalized with borderline symptoms. As prospective studies, they identified a group of individuals (a **cohort**) with borderline symptoms or a diagnosis of BPD and observed them over time to monitor any changes in status that may occur. There may or may not have been a control (or comparison) group of individuals with a different treatment or disorder. The advantages of prospective studies are that they begin with baseline observations and are not affected by recall bias.

● ● ●

Only large-scale, long-term prospective studies of the course of BPD will permit a naturalistic assessment of the outcome and the factors most closely associated with improvement or lack of improvement.

● ● ●

In the first of these early studies, Grinker and associates (1968) studied 41 patients at a mean of 2.5 years after hospitalization and found that two-thirds of the patients described themselves as worse off, the same, or only marginally improved since their hospitalization. Although one-third required rehospitalization during the follow-up period, the majority were occupationally stable but working in low-level jobs. Their social functioning was comparatively more impaired, with most having limited leisure-time activities and transient contact with people. Nearly half of the patients had troubled or minimal relationships with their families. Werble (1970) published a 6- to 7-year follow-up of 28 of the same patients and found that most lived in the community; about half had been rehospitalized, but only briefly. They continued to work but were socially isolated, having little contact with either family or friends.

Gunderson and his colleagues (1975) studied the 2-year course of a group of 24 patients given a borderline diagnosis who were matched by age, sex, race, and socioeconomic status with 29 schizophrenic patients. The researchers found that, on average, these patients had been employed part- to full-time for much of the year prior to follow-up, had social contacts about every other week, and had been hospitalized for less than 3 months during the previous year. Their signs and symptoms were described as both moderate and intermittent. In every area, the borderline patients remained as functionally impaired as the schizophrenic control group.

Carpenter and Gunderson (1977) followed up with 14 of the original 24 patients 5 years after diagnosis. The patients' functioning was still indistinguishable from that of the schizophrenic group, except that the borderline patients maintained the quality of their social contacts, whereas those of the schizophrenic patients deteriorated. Relatively few had required hospitalization. Although several were "loners," most met regularly with friends. Almost all patients were employed continuously, although some were underemployed. Overall, their functioning had not changed significantly since their 2-year follow-up.

Studies Conducted in the 1980s

The studies conducted during the 1980s reflected the use of the newly published *DSM*-III (American Psychiatric Association 1980) *diagnostic criteria* developed to describe borderline symptoms. These studies examined the occurrence of *comorbid* (coexisting) disorders, including alcohol and substance abuse, rates of rehospitalization, and occupational and social functioning. Pope and associates (1983) applied the new criteria retrospectively to a group of patients by reviewing their medical records. These researchers followed up 27 of 33 patients with BPD as defined by DSM-III for 4–7 years after their first hospitalization. Two-thirds of these patients had a probable or definite diagnosis of BPD at follow-up. As a whole, the group of patients with BPD had a significantly worse outcome than control groups with bipolar or schizoaffective disorders. They were similar to a schizophrenia control group on most outcome indices, except that the BPD patients had significantly better occupational functioning.

Pope and colleagues (1983) were also the first to study comorbid diagnoses of borderline patients and their effect on outcome. They compared patients with "pure" BPD with those having a concurrent major *affective* (or mood) disorder and found that BPD patients with the affective disorder were functioning better socially and had fewer symptoms. The researchers linked this finding to the fact that these patients were more likely to have had a positive response to medication.

Akiskal and co-workers (1985) also studied the occurrence of *mood disorders* in BPD and found that one-half of the 100 outpatients with BPD they observed over a period of 6 months to 3 years developed mood disorders during the follow-up period. These included major depression, *manic* episodes, *hypomanic* episodes, and mixed affective disorders. Many of these patients had a diagnosis of concurrent mood disorder at the beginning of the study, but even in the group that had no initial diagnosis of affective disorder, 11 patients had an episode of major depression, and 4 committed suicide. These investigators hypothesized that borderline personality might represent an atypical form of bipolar disorder.

Also in 1985, Barasch and colleagues conducted a 3-year follow-up of 10 patients with BPD diagnosed according to DSM-III diagnostic criteria and a reference group of 20 patients with other DSM-III personality disorders. These researchers found that the two groups were similar in their functioning and the slight degree of their improvement over the follow-up period. Forty percent in each group developed a major depressive episode during the follow-up period. Therefore, neither the degree of their impairment nor their level of affective symptoms distinguished the two groups. In addition, these researchers assessed the degree of stability of the borderline diagnosis over the follow-up period. Sixty percent of the BPD group met DSM-III criteria for BPD at follow-up, and 30% met four (rather than five) DSM-III criteria. Of the 20 nonborderline subjects, only three met DSM-III criteria for BPD at follow-up. The authors concluded that BPD was a stable diagnosis over time and that it was neither a variant of major depression nor a nonspecific label for severe personality disorders.

Perry and Cooper (1985) compared a group of 30 borderline patients with a group of patients diagnosed as having antisocial personality disorder according to DSM-III diagnostic criteria and a group of patients with bipolar II disorder 1–3 years after their initial assessment. The researchers used a semistructured diagnostic interview to assess the presence of BPD by DSM-III criteria. With regard to *global functioning,* these investigators found that the mean score on the *Global Assessment Scale (GAS;* Endicott et al. 1976) for their BPD group was 51, which is considered to be in the "fair" range. They also found no differences on this measure among their three groups at 2- to 3-year follow-up. However, borderline pathology was predictive of both lower GAS scores and greater variability in functioning. During the follow-up period, Perry and Cooper found several differences between patients with BPD and those with antisocial personality disorder. They found that the patients with BPD used significantly more psychiatric health services (after controlling for gender) and that borderline patients without antisocial pathology were more depressed and anxious.

Nace and colleagues (1986) studied 59 alcoholic inpatients diagnosed by using the criteria of the original *Diagnostic Interview for Borderlines* (DIB; Gunderson et al. 1981). Thirteen met criteria for BPD and were found to have a significant decrease in their use of alcohol at 1-year follow-up, a significant improvement in satisfaction with their home and family situation as well as their use of leisure time, and a significant decrease in their number of hospitalizations. Compared with nonborderline alcoholic patients, those with BPD were significantly more likely to be using drugs (but not alcohol) during the follow-up year. They were also significantly more likely to be working and significantly less likely to have a good relationship with their parents.

Tucker and colleagues (1987) studied 40 patients with "borderline disorders"—not DSM-III BPD—who were hospitalized on a specialized long-term treatment unit. Two years after discharge, these patients had less suicidal *ideation* and behavior, were more likely to be in continuous psychotherapy, and had more close friendships and positive relationships than at baseline. Those hospitalized for more than 12 months were less likely to be rehospitalized and were more likely to be in continuous psychotherapy during the first year after discharge, but these differences disappeared after the first year. The mean GAS scores for this sample were 29.7 at admission, 41.6 at discharge, 50.3 one year after discharge, and 56.5 two years after discharge, indicating that these patients moved from the "incapacitated" to the "fair" range of functioning.

In 1989, Modestin and Villiger compared Swiss patients with BPD to Swiss patients with other personality disorders. After observing 18 patients diagnosed with BPD according to DSM-III criteria and 17 patients with diagnoses of heterogeneous nonborderline personality disorders for 4½ years, the authors found that patients with BPD were quite impaired, with about 70% only working part time or receiving a disability pension. However, these patients functioned at about the same vocational and social level as the control group, with the exception that significantly fewer were married. These investigators also found that patients with BPD were more often re-hospitalized, but their hospitalizations were of shorter duration. However, both groups exhibited the same high level of depressive and anxiety symptoms.

Small Studies During the 1990s

The small studies from the 1990s were mainly conducted in Canada and Northern Europe and focused on social and occupational functioning, the stability of the BPD diagnosis over time, and participation in various outpatient treatments. Links and his associates (1990) studied 88 Canadian inpatients diagnosed with BPD by the DIB and found that 40% of the 65 subjects who were reinterviewed 2 years after their first admission no longer met these criteria. They also found that 20% of their borderline subjects were employed full time for the entire follow-up period, 83% had weekly contact with friends, 60% were hospitalized for less than 5% of the follow-up period, and 69% were in continuous outpatient treatment for about a year. At the time of the second follow-up (Links et al. 1995, 1998), these investigators found that patients in the study group who were symptomatic were significantly more likely than those in remission to have major depression, *dysthymia,* and other *Axis II* disorders, particularly the anxious cluster of personality disorders. These patients also had significantly more episodes of substance abuse and dependence than those in remission and were more dependent on disability payments than those in remission.

Mehlum and colleagues (1991) studied 34 day-hospital patients in Norway who received a clinical diagnosis of BPD. When 25 of these patients were reassessed 2–5 years later, their overall scores on the *Health-Sickness Rating Scale* (HSRS; Luborsky 1962) rose from a mean of 39 to a mean of 49—a significant improvement but still in the marginal range of functioning. More than half were employed, 39% were self-supporting, and 48% had been hospitalized (during a mean of 11% of the follow-up period). In addition, these 25 patients had spent 41% of the follow-up period in therapy and 32% of the time on medication.

In an Australian study, Stevenson and Meares (1992) observed 30 outpatients enrolled in an intensive course of standardized psychotherapy. All 30 met DSM-III criteria for BPD at baseline, but 30% had experienced a remission by the time the 12-month treatment program had ended.

Linehan and associates (1993) studied 39 women with DIB-diagnosed BPD 1 year after they had finished a year of randomized treatment with either *dialectical behavior therapy (DBT)* or treatment as usual. The DBT group had significantly fewer episodes of *parasuicidal behavior* at 18 months (but not 24 months) than those in the comparison group.

In addition to social functioning, the next two studies examined the use of medications in the groups of patients observed. Sandell and associates (1993) studied 132 broadly defined borderline patients in day treatment in Sweden. They followed up on 86 patients 3–10 years later through a mailed questionnaire and found that 26% were engaged in full-time work, 34% were receiving disability, 26% were married or living with partners, and 47% were living alone. The investigators also found that 12% of patients had been prescribed *anxiolytics;* 29% had been prescribed *neuroleptics;* and 6% had been prescribed antidepressants.

Antikainen and co-workers (1995) studied 62 broadly defined borderline patients who had been treated on a long-term inpatient unit in Finland designed especially for patients with BPD. Forty-two patients participated in the follow-up interview 3 years later. Sixty-four percent had been unable to work for at least 1 year, and 33% were currently married. Forty-five percent had been hospitalized, 52% were in therapy, 67% had been prescribed anxiolytics, 40% had been prescribed neuroleptics, and 52% had been prescribed antidepressants.

● ● ●

> *Small-scale studies have shown that border-line patients continued to have substantial difficulty 6 months to 7 years after their initial assessment, particularly in the areas of social functioning and the need for continuing psychiatric care.*

● ● ●

Najavits and Gunderson (1995) observed 37 female inpatients diagnosed with the DIB who were beginning a new psychotherapy. Thirty-three were reinterviewed 1 year after their induction into the study, 23 were reinterviewed 2 years after this admission, and 20 were reinterviewed 3 years after their first admission. Their GAS scores increased from a mean of 44 at baseline to 57 at reinterview 3 years later, indicating that as a group the remaining subjects moved from the "marginal" to the "fair" range of functioning.

Senol and colleagues (1997) studied 61 clinically diagnosed borderline inpatients in Turkey, 45 of whom consented to a follow-up interview 2–4 years after their index admission. Their mean GAS score increased from 41 to 46, a statistically significant but clinically minor difference. It was also found that only 4% experienced a remission of their BPD but that 54% had had a mood disorder and 56% had had a substance use disorder during the follow-up period.

Lessons Learned From These Studies

The *generalizability* of the results of these studies has been limited by a number of methodological problems. These problems include small sample sizes, high *attrition* rates, the absence of comparison groups or the use of psychotic comparison groups, lack of explicit criteria for BPD, the use of unstructured assessment techniques for making diagnoses, non-*blinded* assessment of outcome status, limited assessment of outcome functioning, varying length of follow-up within the same study, and only one follow-up wave for most of the studies.

Despite these limitations, three major findings concerning the short-term course of BPD have emerged from these studies. First, borderline patients continued to have substantial difficulty functioning 6 months to 7 years after their initial assessment, particularly in the areas of social functioning and the need for continuing psychiatric care. Second, their level of functioning was very similar to that of patients with both schizophrenia and other forms of personality disorder. Third, BPD patients did not go on to develop schizophrenia but retained the chronic instability characteristic of a borderline diagnosis.

Large-Scale, Long-Term Follow-Back Studies of the Course of BPD

Follow-back (or retrospective) studies have the advantage of using treatment records to diagnose large numbers of patients with a particular diagnosis. However, a major disadvantage is that researchers can make few predictions about the course of the disorder and its treatments going forward. In the first of these large-scale studies, Plakun and associates (1985) conducted a follow-back study of 237 patients who had been hospitalized between 1950 and 1976 at Austin Riggs, a private psychiatric hospital in western Massachusetts. The investigators had originally mailed out a 50-item questionnaire to the 878 patients who had been hospitalized for at least 2 months, and they received responses from 27% of the patients (another potential drawback to this type of study). Among those diagnosed through chart review according to DSM-III criteria were the following patient groups: 61 BPD patients, 19 schizophrenic patients, 24 patients with major affective disorder, 13 schizotypal patients, and 19 patients with schizoid personality disorder. At a mean follow-up period of 15 years, the borderline patients achieved a mean GAS score of 67, which is in the "good" range of functioning. Both the 54 "aggregated" borderline patients (all but those with a coexisting major mood disorder) and the borderline patients with a comorbid schizotypal disorder achieved a higher mean GAS score than the schizophrenic patients. In addition, borderline patients without a comorbid affective disorder were functioning significantly better than those who also had a mood disorder.

In the second large-scale study, McGlashan (1986) followed up all inpatients treated at Chestnut Lodge Hospital in Rockville, Maryland, between 1950 and 1975 who met the following criteria: 1) index admission of at least 90 days; 2) age between 16 and 55; and 3) absence of an organic brain syndrome. Follow-up information was obtained on 446 patients, resulting in a trace rate of 72%, and was collected by the use of a *semistructured clinical interview* by telephone with the patient or an informant. Most comparisons focused on 81 patients meeting criteria for BPD only, 163 who met criteria for schizophrenia, and 44 who met criteria for major depression, with diagnoses being derived through retrospective chart review.

● ● ●

These large-scale follow-back studies show that the functioning of borderline patients over time is highly variable. Some function very well, many continue to have substantial difficulty in a number of areas of their lives, and 3%–10% commit suicide.

● ● ●

McGlashan found that his borderline patients achieved an overall HSRS score of 64 a mean of 15 years after their first admission (range 2–32 years). This mean rating represents a good level of functioning and was equal to that of depressed control subjects but significantly higher than that of schizophrenic patients. However, closer examination reveals that although half of the borderline patients (53%) were functioning in the "good–recovered" range, the other half (47%) were functioning in the "moderate–incapacitated" range. In addition, 3% of the traced borderline patients had committed suicide. In terms of instrumental functioning, those with BPD worked about half the time at reasonably complex jobs. They also met with friends about once every other week. About half were married or living with a sexual partner, and about half avoided intimate relationships entirely. In terms of further treatment, the average borderline patient was rehospitalized one or two more times, spending about 8% of the follow-up period as an inpatient. They used psychosocial treatments during about one-third of the follow-up period (35%) and *psychotropic medications* about one-fourth of the time (22%). Almost half (46%) were receiving some form of psychiatric treatment at the time of their follow-up interview. These figures were very similar to those achieved by the depressed control subjects. However, the borderline patients functioned significantly better than schizophrenic patients in the instrumental realm and used significantly less psychiatric treatment than these comparison subjects with a psychotic disorder.

McGlashan found that overall functioning was significantly related to the length of the follow-up period. He found that patients who were followed up for 10–19 years had significantly better overall functioning than those observed for 9 years or less and about the same level of functioning as those studied for 20 years or more. He also found that overall functioning of these patients over time followed the pattern of an inverted U, with functioning improving through their 20s and 30s, peaking in their 40s, and declining in their 50s.

In their study, Paris and colleagues (1987) reviewed the charts of all patients hospitalized for psychiatric reasons at the Jewish General Hospital in Montreal between 1958 and 1978. Retrospective analysis showed that 322 patients met DIB criteria for BPD, and 100 of these patients (31.5%) were reinterviewed a mean of 15 years after their first admission. The researchers found that all aspects of the patients' borderline psychopathology as measured by a live DIB interview had decreased significantly. The investigators also found that only 25% of these patients still met DIB criteria for BPD. In terms of overall functioning, these borderline patients achieved a mean HSRS score of 63, indicating a good global outcome. They also achieved a mean work score of 3.8, indicating frequent job changes without unemployment. Their social participation score was 3.2, close to a level described as limited leisure time with transient social contact. In terms of further treatment, they had a mean of 1.3 rehospitalizations and a mean of 1.9 years of further treatment. Overall, there was great variability in the amount of treatment received, but most of the patients' treatment histories were chaotic and intermittent. Of the 165 patients who could be located or tracked, 14 (8.5%) had committed suicide.

Paris and Zweig-Frank (2001) later reassessed this sample of patients once diagnosed as borderline a mean of 27 years after their first admission. The researchers found that of the 64 inpatients interviewed, only 5 (7.8%) met the particularly restrictive Revised Diagnostic Interview for Borderlines (DIB-R) criteria for BPD (Zanarini et al. 1989). In addition, 83% had been married or had lived with a partner at some point, and 59% had children. However, the mean *Global Assessment of Functioning (GAF)* score for these patients still had not progressed to the "recovered" range, and 10.3% of the original borderline cohort had committed suicide by the time of the second follow-up assessment.

In the last of these large-scale studies, Stone (1990) followed up 502 (91%) of the 550 patients hospitalized at the New York State Psychiatric Institute between 1963 and 1976 meeting the following inclusion criteria: 1) a stay of at least 3 months; 2) age under 40 years; and 3) IQ of 90 or higher. Most of these patients were selected for their potential to benefit from intensive psychotherapy. However, a substantial minority were admitted because of their family's social status. Stone made retrospective DSM-III diagnoses after reviewing each patient's chart, and he then attempted to contact each patient, most of whom he had known during their first hospitalization. He was able to trace 193 (94%) of the 206 patients meeting DSM-III criteria for BPD, and he interviewed relatives or other informants when patients were unavailable. Stone found that the average GAS score of this group of patients a mean of 16 years after their index admission was 67. This score, which indicates a good level of functioning, was significantly higher than that achieved by schizophrenic comparison subjects. Almost half of the surviving borderline patients received a GAS score in the "recovered" range (41%), 28% received a score in the "good" range, 18% were in the "fair" range, and 13% were in the "marginal–incapacitated" range. This distribution was also significantly different from that attained by the schizophrenic patients in the study, with only 6% of these patients receiving GAS scores in the "recovered" range.

In terms of more specific spheres of follow-up functioning, 53% of the borderline patients had worked at least three-quarters of the time, 17% had worked about half the time, and 30% worked less than half the time or not at all. Fewer than half (45%) had ever married, and fewer than a quarter (23%) had children. However, only 28% had ever been rehospitalized or had spent time in another institution. In addition, borderline patients functioned better in each of these spheres than schizophrenic patients. Despite these generally optimistic findings, it is important to note that 8.8% of the BPD patients diagnosed according to DSM-III criteria committed suicide, a rate similar to that found for schizophrenic patients (9.4%) but substantially lower than that found for patients with schizoaffective disorder (23%).

Lessons Learned From the Follow-Back Studies

Despite the consistency of the findings in these four studies, the generalizability of their results is limited by a number of methodological problems. These problems include the use of highly variable chart material as the basis for diagnoses; assessment of posthospital functioning at only one point in time in three of the four studies; absence of detailed information concerning follow-up functioning; use of mailed questionnaires or telephone interviews as the only or the primary source of information; use of upper middle class inpatient samples from tertiary facilities; lack of independence of baseline and follow-up data; absence of comparison subjects or failure to use near-neighbor Axis II comparison subjects; the wide range of follow-up periods in each study; and the presence of different age cohorts.

Despite these limitations, one major finding has emerged from these studies: that the functioning of borderline patients over time is highly variable. Some function very well, many continue to have substantial difficulty in a number of areas of their lives, and 3%–10% commit suicide.

Large-Scale, Long-Term Prospective Studies of the Course of BPD

Large-scale, long-term prospective studies combine the strengths of each of the other study designs and offer the best hope for making predictions about the course of BPD and the success of its treatments over time. The National Institute of Mental Health (NIMH) has funded two large-scale prospective studies of the longitudinal course of borderline personality disorder. One of these studies, the McLean Study of Adult Development (MSAD), began 12 years ago. A second study, the Collaborative Longitudinal Personality Disorders Study (CLPS), began 8 years ago.

McLean Study of Adult Development

Zanarini and her colleagues' (2003) MSAD study began with a sample of 362 patients with personality disorders. All of these women and men were initially inpatients at McLean Hospital in Belmont, Massachusetts, who were admitted during a 3-year period (1992–1995). Each patient was initially screened to determine that he or she 1) was between ages 18 and 35; 2) had a known or estimated IQ of 71 or higher; 3) had no history or current symptoms of an organic condition that could cause psychiatric symptoms, schizophrenia, schizoaffective disorder, or bipolar I disorder; and 4) was fluent in English. After a careful diagnostic assessment involving three semistructured clinical interviews of proven reliability, 290 patients were found to meet both DIB-R and DSM-III-R (American Psychiatric Association 1987) criteria for BPD. The other 72 patients were found to meet criteria for another form of Axis II disorder (and neither criteria set for BPD).

Three 2-year waves of follow-up interviews have been completed. More than 94% of the surviving members of the original sample were re-interviewed at all three of these follow-up periods. Three important findings concerning the symptomatic course of BPD have emerged from this study. The first is that remissions of BPD were found to be more common than was previously known. More specifically, 34.5% of patients who received diagnoses of BPD no longer met study criteria for BPD at 2-year follow-up; 49.4% no longer met the criteria at 4-year follow-up; 68.6% no longer met the criteria at 6-year follow-up; and 73.5% no longer met the criteria at one or more of the follow-up periods.

The second important finding concerning the symptomatic status of BPD is that these remissions were quite stable, and therefore recurrences were quite rare. In fact, only 6% of borderline patients who had experienced a remission had a symptomatic resurgence that qualified as a recurrence of BPD.

The third important symptom-related finding of the MSAD study was that all of the 24 symptoms of BPD that were studied declined significantly over time, but 23 of the 24 remained significantly more common among those with BPD than among the Axis II comparison subjects. However, it was found that the four core symptom areas of BPD did not decline at an equal rate. Affective symptoms declined the least, and *impulsive* symptoms declined the most. It was also found that *cognitive* and interpersonal symptoms occupied an intermediate position in terms of symptom reduction over time.

Zanarini and her colleagues heuristically described some symptoms as acute and others as temperamental. Symptoms of the first type tend to resolve relatively rapidly, have been found to be excellent markers for BPD (Zanarini et al. 1990), and are often the most pressing reason for psychiatric hospitalization. These acute symptoms include self-mutilative acts, help-seeking suicidal efforts, and quasi-psychotic thought. The second group of symptoms tended to be nonspecific to BPD and also tended to resolve quite slowly. Among these symptoms are chronic feelings of anger and angry acts, stormy relationships, and concerns about abandonment.

It should be noted that the MSAD sample is a heavily treated sample, with more than 70% of the patients with BPD still in psychotherapy and still taking psychotropic medication 6 years after their first admission. It should also be noted that the study has a low suicide rate of 3.8% ($n=11$). The reasons for this unexpectedly low suicide rate are unclear, but Zanarini and Frankenburg (1994) have speculated that the more supportive, trauma-sensitive psychotherapy that many patients are receiving may be better suited to their "hyperbolic" temperaments and their personal histories.

Collaborative Longitudinal Study of Personality Disorders

The CLPS study used a well-established semistructured diagnostic interview to make baseline Axis II diagnoses (Shea et al. 2002). Of the study's 668 subjects, 158 had a primary diagnosis of BPD. Of these 668 subjects— all of whom were in treatment, had a treatment history, or were seeking psychiatric treatment—93% were reinterviewed at 6 and 12 months after their baseline assessment. These follow-along assessments were conducted by using a modified version of the same diagnostic interview, which assesses Axis II criteria on a monthly basis. At the end of 1 year of follow-along assessment, which was typically not blinded, 59% of the borderline subjects did not meet five or more criteria for BPD for each of the 12 months assessed. In fact, most of the change occurred during the 6 months immediately after their induction into the study.

● ● ●

Taken together, the results from two method-ologically rigorous studies cast a more positive light on the course of BPD than did earlier studies.

● ● ●

The reasons for the more rapid rate of "remissions" in the CLPS than in the MSAD study are unclear. It may be that the MSAD subjects were more severely ill, since all of them were inpatients at the time that their study participation began. It may also be more difficult to drop below threshold on two different criteria sets than on only one, particularly because the DIB-R has a complicated weighted scoring system that defines a smaller subset of patients as having BPD (Zanarini et al. 1989).

Conclusion

Taken together, the results of these two methodologically rigorous studies cast a more positive light on the course of BPD than did earlier studies. Further reports from these studies will delineate the psychosocial functioning of borderline patients over time; the predictive factors associated with remission of BPD; and, ultimately, recovery from this most troubling and misunderstood disorder.

What Families Need to Know

Key Messages in This Chapter

- Little is known about the long-term outlook for individuals with BPD and why some people with the disorder make progress and others do not.
- Compared with the large number of studies examining the longitudinal course of schizophrenia or bipolar disorder, very few studies have followed the course of BPD over time.
- Despite their limitations, the early small-scale studies of the course of BPD found that patients have difficulty functioning socially as long as 7 years after diagnosis and continue to need psychiatric care.

- Follow-back (or retrospective) studies of larger groups of patients identified through their treatment records have shown that the course of BPD is highly variable over time; some patients function well in work and social situations, whereas others struggle, and 3%–10% commit suicide.
- The two long-term prospective studies of the course of BPD currently under way have had differing results. The McLean Study of Adult Development (MSAD) found that remission of borderline symptoms was common but that affective symptoms declined more slowly than impulsivity. The Collaborative Longitudinal Study of Personality Disorders (CLPS) found a faster rate of remission in the BPD patients they studied: at 1-year follow-up, more than half did not meet criteria for BPD.
- These more rigorous studies suggest a more positive outlook for individuals with BPD and their families. Further reports from these ongoing studies will examine the factors associated with remission and may offer new hope for recovery.

Key Words in This Chapter

affective   pertaining to one's emotional state.

anxiolytics   medications that reduce anxiety.

attrition   the rate of dropout among subjects in a follow-up study.

Axis I   a classification in DSM-IV-TR (American Psychiatric Association 2000) consisting of major psychiatric disorders, including mood disorders (depression and bipolar disorder), anxiety disorders, eating disorders, schizophrenia, etc.

Axis II   a classification in DSM-IV-TR for personality disorders, for example, BPD.

blinded   a type of study in which the raters are not aware of the initial diagnostic status or level of functioning of subjects in the study.

cognitive   referring to thinking or reasoning.

cohort   a group of similar individuals studied over time.

comorbid   occurring together with another disease or condition.

diagnostic criteria   a list of clinical features that must be present for the diagnosis of a mental disorder to be made.

Diagnostic Interview for Borderlines (DIB)   an interview designed by Gunderson and Zanarini to diagnose BPD.

dialectical behavior therapy (DBT)   a treatment for BPD developed by Marsha Linehan combining aspects of cognitive and behavioral therapy. The treatment teaches specific skills to manage emotions, control impulsiveness, and diminish self-destructive behavior.

DSM *Diagnostic and Statistical Manual of Mental Disorders;* the American system of classification of psychiatric diagnoses.

dysthymia a chronic low-grade depression.

follow-back (retrospective) studies studies in which subjects are generally identified by medical records as having a particular diagnosis, then followed back in time to look for associations with that diagnosis.

generalizability the degree to which results of a study can be applied to a larger population.

Global Assessment of Functioning (GAF) a scale used by clinicians to judge patients' overall social, occupational, and psychological functioning over a specific time period.

Global Assessment Scale (GAS) a revised version of the Health-Sickness Rating Scale (HSRS).

global functioning overall social, occupational, and psychological functioning.

Health-Sickness Rating Scale (HSRS) the first rating scale of overall psychological health describing symptoms and level of functioning; provides an overall rating on a scale of 0–100.

hypomanic an abnormally elevated mood and level of bodily activity (restlessness) leading to some interference with daily living.

ideation thoughts or formation of ideas.

impulsivity inability to resist performing some action.

manic characterized by excessive excitement, elevated mood, and grandiosity.

mood disorders a group of disorders (including depression and bipolar disorder) in which a disturbance of mood is accompanied by impaired cognitive function and physical signs, such as disturbed sleep, changes in appetite, and lack of energy.

neuroleptics antipsychotic medications.

parasuicidal behavior any self-injurious behavior, with or without suicidal intent, that does not result in death.

prognosis prediction about the future course of a condition, including the chance for remission or relapse.

prospective study a research design following a group of subjects forward in time.

psychotropic medications all drugs that affect psychological function, behavior, or experience.

semistructured clinical interview an interview that requires probing to elicit needed information.

References

Akiskal HS, Chen SE, Davis GC, et al: Borderline: an adjective in search of a noun. J Clin Psychiatry 46:41–48, 1985

American Psychiatric Association: Diagnostic and Statistical Manual of Mental Disorders, 3rd Edition. Washington, DC, American Psychiatric Association, 1980

American Psychiatric Association: Diagnostic and Statistical Manual of Mental Disorders, 3rd Edition, Revised. Washington, DC, American Psychiatric Association, 1987

American Psychiatric Association: Diagnostic and Statistical Manual of Mental Disorders, 4th Edition, Text Revision. Washington, DC, American Psychiatric Association, 2000

Antikainen R, Hintikka J, Lehtonen J, et al: A prospective three-year follow-up study of borderline personality disorder inpatients. Acta Psychiatr Scand 92:327–335, 1995

Barasch A, Frances A, Hurt S, et al: The stability and distinctness of borderline personality disorder. Am J Psychiatry 142:1484–1486, 1985

Carpenter WT, Gunderson JG: Five year follow-up comparison of borderline and schizophrenic patients. Compr Psychiatry 18:567–571, 1977

Endicott J, Spitzer RL, Fleiss JL, et al: The Global Assessment Scale: a procedure for measuring overall severity of psychiatric disturbance. Arch Gen Psychiatry 33:766–771, 1976

Grinker RR, Werble B, Drye RC: The Borderline Syndrome: A Behavioral Study of Ego-Functions. New York, Basic Books, 1968

Gunderson JG, Carpenter WT, Strauss JS: Borderline and schizophrenic patients: a comparative study. Am J Psychiatry 132:1257–1264, 1975

Gunderson JG, Kolb JE, Austin V: The diagnostic interview for borderline patients. Am J Psychiatry 138:896–903, 1981

Linehan MM, Heard HL, Armstrong HF: Naturalistic follow-up of a behavioral treatment for chronically parasuicidal borderline patients. Arch Gen Psychiatry 50:971–974, 1993

Links PS, Mitton JE, Steiner M: Predicting outcome for borderline personality disorder. Compr Psychiatry 31:490–498, 1990

Links PS, Heslegrave RJ, Mitton JE, et al: Borderline psychopathology and recurrences of clinical disorders. J Nerv Ment Dis 183:582–586, 1995

Links PS, Heslegrave RJ, Van Reekum R: Prospective follow-up study of borderline personality disorder: prognosis, prediction of outcome, and Axis II comorbidity. Can J Psychiatry 42:265–270, 1998

Luborsky L: Clinician's judgments of mental health: a proposed scale. Arch Gen Psychiatry 7:407–417, 1962

McGlashan TH: The Chestnut Lodge follow-up study, III: long-term outcome of borderline personalities. Arch Gen Psychiatry 43:20–30, 1986

Mehlum L, Friis S, Irion T, et al: Personality disorders 2–5 years after treatment: a prospective follow-up study. Acta Psychiatr Scand 84:72–77, 1991

Modestin J, Villiger C: Follow-up study on borderline versus nonborderline disorders. Compr Psychiatry 30:236–244, 1989

Nace EP, Saxon JJ, Shore N: Borderline personality disorder and alcoholism treatment: a one-year follow-up study. J Stud Alcohol 47:196–200, 1986

Najavits LM, Gunderson JG: Better than expected: improvements in borderline personality disorder in a 3-year prospective outcome study. Compr Psychiatry 36:296–302, 1995

Paris J, Zweig-Frank H: A 27-year follow-up of patients with borderline personality disorder. Compr Psychiatry 42:482–487, 2001

Paris J, Brown R, Nowlis D: Long-term follow-up of borderline patients in a general hospital. Compr Psychiatry 28:530–535, 1987

Perry J, Cooper S: Psychodynamic symptoms and outcome in borderline and antisocial personality disorders and bipolar II affective disorder, in The Borderline: Current Empirical Research. Washington, DC, American Psychiatric Press, 1985, pp 9–41

Plakun EM, Burkhardt PE, Muller JP: 14-year follow-up of borderline and schizotypal personality disorders. Compr Psychiatry 26:448–455, 1985

Pope HG, Jonas JM, Hudson JI, et al: The validity of DSM-III borderline personality disorder: a phenomenologic, family history, treatment response, and long-term follow-up study. Arch Gen Psychiatry 40:23–30, 1983

Sandell R, Alfredsson E, Berg M, et al: Clinical significance of outcome in long-term follow-up of borderline patients at a day hospital. Acta Psychiatr Scand 87:405–413, 1993

Senol S, Dereboy C, Yuksel N: Borderline disorder in Turkey: a 2- to 4-year follow-up. Soc Psychiatry Psychiatr Epidemiol 32:109–112, 1997

Shea MT, Stout R, Gunderson J, et al: Short-term diagnostic stability of schizotypal, borderline, avoidant, and obsessive-compulsive personality disorders. Am J Psychiatry 159:2036–2041, 2002

Stevenson J, Meares R: An outcome study of psychotherapy for patients with borderline personality disorder. Am J Psychiatry 149:358–362, 1992

Stone MH: The Fate of Borderline Patients. New York, Guilford, 1990

Tucker L, Bauer SF, Wagner S, et al: Long-term hospital treatment of borderline patients: a descriptive outcome study. Am J Psychiatry 144:1443–1448, 1987

Werble B: Second follow-up study of borderline patients. Arch Gen Psychiatry 23:1–7, 1970

Zanarini MC, Frankenburg FR: Emotional hypochondriasis, hyperbole, and the borderline patient. J Psychother Pract Res 3:25–36, 1994

Zanarini MC, Gunderson JG, Frankenburg FR, et al: The Revised Diagnostic Interview for Borderlines: discriminating BPD from other Axis II disorders. J Personal Disord 3:10–18, 1989

Zanarini MC, Gunderson JG, Frankenburg FR, et al: Discriminating borderline personality disorder from other Axis II disorders. Am J Psychiatry 147:161–167, 1990

Zanarini MC, Frankenburg FR, Hennen J, et al: The longitudinal course of borderline psychopathology: six-year prospective follow-up of the phenomenology of borderline personality disorder. Am J Psychiatry 160:274–283, 2003

Part
II

Family Matters

• 6 •

Living With Borderline Personality Disorder

Two Firsthand Accounts

Anonymous

I.
A Question of Identity

I was 22 when I was diagnosed with borderline personality disorder (BPD). At first I found that having a labeled container for my bewildering grab bag of symptoms was reassuring, even exciting. It almost—but not quite—gave me a sense of identity, and I bought every book I could find with the words *borderline personality* on the cover. Bulimia with occasional bouts of starvation; suicide attempts that were more tantrum than longing for death; binge drinking; and that vague, awful ice-slush-in-the-stomach emptiness that would surround me and seal me off even in a warm, rowdy crowd—it turned out they were all part of the disorder.

Of course, I had never heard of BPD and was unaware of its nasty reputation, so I rushed to tell my parents, who told their doctor, who told them my only hope was that it was a misdiagnosis. But I was just relieved that I wasn't making it all up and malingering, as everybody had begun to suspect. The gravity of the situation had yet to hit me. Besides, I already knew I felt crazy half the time. Everything I did seemed to fall under one or another of the nine diagnostic criteria for BPD. If frantic efforts to avoid abandonment included deciding a friend suddenly despised me—and so never speaking to her again—I had it. I'd always been impulsive (but preferred to refer to it as being into immediate gratification, because that made it sound as if decision was involved), and everything I did was to excess. But wasn't it Colette who said, "If I can't have too many truffles, I don't want any truffles?"

As for identity disturbance, I absolutely didn't know who I was or what I wanted. I didn't even know if I wanted to stay alive badly enough to work at getting better. So much of myself was symptom, but of course it was my personality that was sick.

● ● ●

There was a small, incomplete layer of me that wanted to live, but this other, powerful voice filled my head like a tidal wave and rushed me into hotel rooms, telling me to hurry up and swallow the pills. The good part of me couldn't compete.

● ● ●

I threw myself into therapy, individual and group. I tried every medication available and even tried sleep deprivation through a psychopharmacologist who was willing to try anything at that point. My therapist wanted to help me, but there was an unending, no-light-at-the-end-of-the-tunnel softness and malleability to the situation that made me want to kick and tear at things. This sounds strange, I know, but I experienced most things, especially frustration, at a very visceral level. I made more and more serious and aggressive suicide attempts.

I hated what I was doing. There was a small, incomplete layer of me that wanted to live, but this other, powerful voice filled my head like a tidal wave and rushed me into hotel rooms, telling me to hurry up and swallow the pills. The good part of me couldn't compete.

For a long time I thought of myself as having developed into a borderline personality in high school with my first serious suicide attempt, and of everything that came before that as falling under the "unhappy childhood/weird kid" heading. I've since read in *Personality Disorders in Children and Adolescents,* by Paulina F. Kernberg et al. (2000), that "identity disturbance was considered the single best discriminating item between borderline children, in whom it is present, and neurotic children, in whom it is absent" (p. 138). Suddenly the memories I had of wearing nightgowns to school as fairy princess costumes well into the third grade (at which point a therapist I was seeing told me that if I wanted friends I should stop it), and of changing my name (once to Sam) on a yearly basis became recognizably borderline. Of course, there were other things I'd done as a child that went beyond neurotic. I had thought I could communicate with cats through mental telepathy, had physically defended my little brother from bullies who had yet to bully him, and had stolen other children's lunches from their cubbies in preschool. I distinctly remember lying about that when confronted and feeling cocooned in the lie even though I knew I wasn't believed, but thinking that if I just insisted on it I was safe. My behavior was inappropriate: during the game of statues, regardless of what position I fell into, I pretended to be a prostitute. In fifth grade, while the rest of the class drew friendly forest creatures, I scandalized my teacher and classmates by drawing a picture of a flame-haired woman in a leopard-skin bikini behind bars.

But hadn't I only been reacting to my eccentric, overstimulating, and (at times) traumatizing or even abusive parents? It wasn't really me. I was zany and creative, madcap. "Look at me. Listen to the hilarious things I've done," I would say to my therapist, waving vamp-red, bitten-to-the-quick fingernails in the air. "Aren't I amusing? And when I get drunk, I sing in cabarets!" Like Sally Bowles or Holly Golightly. Of course, there is that part at the end of *Breakfast at Tiffany's* (Capote 1958) when she abandons her cat in an alley, screams at him to scram, and stomps her foot to scare him off. In the book she doesn't go back to find him as she does in the movie, where they're reunited, smiling and tearful in the rain.

● ● ●

I would drag my heels against feelings pulling
me away from a person I had worked toward
having as a friend, a person I didn't want to
hurt. But there was never any going back.

● ● ●

In real life, BPD cost me the chance to kiss the first boy I ever really liked in school. It was May in the arboretum and it had rained the night before. He was tall and very sincere, and he was quite startled at my refusal, as I remember. I always imagined it was the other people who had changed. Something would seem different about the way they looked, and my feelings for them would cloud over like your feelings do when someone is twisted mean and not themselves in a dream the night before. Only you don't remember the dream, and so you can't brush it out of your way to see them now in daylight. I fought it. I would drag my heels against the feeling pulling me away from a person I had worked toward having as a friend, a person I didn't want to hurt. But there was never any going back. I regret all those years spent tossing away friendships. Some of them wouldn't have held up, but I might have a circle of friends today. We'd be at that relaxed, worn-in stage by now, like family, but better for having been chosen. And in real life, I hadn't had the courage to sing in a cabaret in a year. My life had become very small.

I was as frightened of the people I worked with as I had once been of the mean kids at school. I called in sick, and when I was too scared to do that I overdosed. It was easier to float away from all of it. Maybe my husband, whom I'd married when I was 21, would come home in time, maybe not. I went to the hospital looking for the same thing I'd tried to find at the nurse's office in kindergarten when I lay on the cot every day, hoping to be discovered feverish and be doted on. I was going backwards, shrinking, imploding, my mother said. Where once I had been reckless and brazen, now I found myself wondering while talking to people, how long eye contact was supposed to last. I felt as if I had walked into every room with an elbow jutting out and couldn't at all manage the light skimming-of-the-surface conversation that normal people did. I either plunged in too deep within seconds or wandered off all out of focus.

● ● ●

Once I began therapy with him, I stopped making suicide attempts—that was part of our contract, and somehow I knew not to mess it up. The part of me that wanted to have a life saw its chance.

● ● ●

Finally, when I was 26, I was referred to a therapist who practiced transference-focused psychotherapy (TFP), and once I began therapy with him I stopped making suicide attempts—that was part of our contract, and somehow I knew not to mess it up. The part of me that wanted to have a life saw its chance. This time there were walls I could get a foothold on and use to climb out of the cave. Our work together was intense, but he withstood even my strongest and most chaotic feelings, which were kept available in the transference for exploration (whereas they'd previously been shunted off into one or another dangerous form of acting out). In *A Primer of Transference-Focused Psychotherapy for the Borderline Patient* (Yeomans et al. 2002), the authors wrote,

> Therapy is not merely an intellectual experience, although it requires both intelligence and knowledge, but also an emotional experience that requires exposure to, without involvement in, the intense affective world of the patient. A somewhat dramatic metaphor is to compare the therapist to Ulysses who, in order to hear the sirens' call without acting in response to it, had himself tied to the mast of the ship so that he could be exposed to it without responding in turn.

And my therapist was there for me, steadfast, no matter how cleverly I tried to drive the therapy off course and crash into rocks.

It's been almost 8 years, and the borderline part of me has been examined, dismantled, and shrunk down into regular-sized pieces: blinding rage is now anger; overwhelming, gnashing frustration is just frustration. I almost can't remember that emptiness now—the feeling of being down and tired in a washed-out way and wanting desperately to latch onto the thought of something that made me happy, but not being able to think of anything. And I've banished the hyper, overstimulated feeling I used to get when I did something as simple as listen to music. (I once overdosed after listening to the waltz from *Carousel* because it was too beautiful, too intense. I felt as if I were filled with yellow birds that were trying to peck their way outside of me.) I was even able to go back and salvage the odds and ends that I liked from my old self. I had left everything behind for a while out of a fear of not knowing the difference between quirky (and creative) and insane. I don't mind quirky.

The me of 8 years ago would have been so astounded to know about this last thing that I worry it might push my hard-earned happy ending into a totally unbelievable, over-the-top-sounding sort of fireworks display: I have a 4-year-old son now. I never thought I would have a child, but in all of my strongest, sanest moments, I wanted a child more than anything. He enjoys being alive so much, and I'm very grateful that he got the chance.

II.
Learn to Take BPD by the Hand

My difficulties began very early. I remember lying in bed at about age six and being terrified of the voices outside my bedroom window—voices that were planning how to kill me. I lay awake for the rest of the night and trembled. I never forgot that incident and I never shared it with anyone either.

I remember when I was a little older, while visiting my grandmother I got dressed for a "grown-up" dinner. As we walked toward the restaurant, it was decided that we should walk out onto a dock and enjoy the setting sun. I don't know what happened, but I kept walking—right off the end of the dock! My father came in after me in his suit, dress shoes and all. My mother was extremely angry. The next day I was ignored, and I knew that I had done something bad and was not to be forgiven.

I remember at age 11 being in trouble with my mother, who was angrier than I had ever seen her in my life. Suddenly I took a deep breath, retreated into myself, and "split" into two. One part remained facing her, but I protected the other part. I imagined taking my inner self out of my body and placing it in a shoebox that I put on the shelf in the closet. I could "disappear" and come back whenever I wanted, and I didn't even have to have memories. I felt safe in my other world, and I remember going to a room that was soft like cotton, and pink (I loved the color pink then.) No one ever knew. I lived in a world where problems were not permitted, where I was told how and what to feel, where everything was a secret from the neighbors, where mental illness was unheard of. I was coping the best way I knew how, and I was surviving.

●   ●   ●

When I spent time without escaping—in the real world, so to speak—my memories, impulsiveness, and terror of being alone got me into trouble and pushed me into quick-fix ways of coping. Drugs, alcohol, cutting, and suicide attempts: I tried them all.

●   ●   ●

In high school I kept to myself and spent hours practicing facial expressions that portrayed no emotion, practicing "splitting" and being two people. Throughout my adolescent and college years, I mentally drifted in and out of different worlds. The trigger was a stressful event, usually from home. I still didn't let anyone get close to me. It took all my energy to play this game of emotional hide-and-seek, go to school, and deal with my mother. Unfortunately, when I spent time without escaping—in the real world, so to speak—my memories, impulsiveness, and terror of being alone got me into trouble and pushed me into quick-fix ways of coping. Drugs, alcohol, cutting, and suicide attempts: I tried them all, but I never considered introspection, because that was just too dangerous. Gradually, as I matured, I learned that I could keep my inner world and the troubles in my family of origin private and could have a lovely and totally acceptable facade.

After college, I went to work and married. It is both interesting and a mystery to me how the man I married was able to walk through my fortress. He never judged me, was kind and respectful, and convinced me that he was interested in who I was, not what the family I had come from was like (although he had my mother pegged as abusive shortly after meeting her). He helped me believe more in myself, and I believed that he and I could walk hand in hand through life; after 26 years I still know that that we love and respect each other deeply. Of course, I still had issues, but he gave me strength. I didn't foresee the problems brewing from my not caring about who I was, as a result of never having developed a self-identity.

● ● ●

The most important thing I have to share is not that I have BPD, but that I now lead a healthy and happy life, a life filled with joys and sorrows, accomplishments and challenges, calm moments and distressful moments.

● ● ●

I went on to have children, and I thought I was lucky to know exactly the kind of mother I didn't want to be. Troubles that I had with my identity regularly surfaced, but I could always "split." However, as I went through my days doing volunteer work or whatever, I often wondered if anyone could see in my eyes what was behind the smile. Ultimately, it didn't matter; life was wonderful.

After the death of my mother, the delicate balance that had held my life together crumbled. Once again I became suspicious, suicidal, and recklessly impulsive. In those dark and chaotic days, I regularly dissociated because I couldn't stand the emptiness, fear, and self-hatred I was experiencing. I was sure that my family would walk out on me if they really knew about me. My behaviors became increasingly dangerous; and I grew more distant from reality. Of course, my family isn't blind or stupid, and they could see I was in trouble.

I was ultimately diagnosed with BPD. It was a crushing blow. It was frightening to feel so out of control, frightening not to understand the diagnosis, frightening not to be able to tell my husband what was wrong, and frightening not to know how to ask the questions that would give us the information we so desperately needed. I was confused. Hadn't I done a good job keeping everything under control? Wasn't I keeping everything in separate boxes that I carefully controlled? Was I a bad girl again?

My mother had died. Why did I feel that I had lost my war with her?

However, the most important thing I have to share is not that I have BPD, but that I now lead a healthy and happy life, a life filled with joys and sorrows, accomplishments and challenges, calm moments and distressful moments. My life isn't an easy life to live, because it can be hard to live in my skin. But I have found that when certain factors are in place, someone with BPD can learn to manage life successfully.

As I see it, four critical and interrelated factors have made it possible for me to learn to live with BPD. The first and most important factor is the willingness to change my way of thinking. Without this commitment to change, nothing can or will happen. It took me 2–3 years after my diagnosis to even acknowledge that I needed to change. Even though I was in therapy during this time, I made little progress. I wouldn't give up my quick-fix behaviors. I was unwilling to tolerate the uncomfortable feelings associated with facing the world in a new way. I am sure that commitment to change can happen faster for some people, but it took me a while to realize that the environment and my memories weren't going to do the changing for me. I had to embrace change and be stubborn in my clumsy attempts to change my behavior. When I realized that I had to change from within, my recovery began in earnest.

The second factor is the involvement of a committed medical team that is there to support you, come hell or high water, and that supplies information in nonthreatening, nontechnical terms. The team might include a therapist, a psychiatrist, a psychopharmacologist, and a nutritionist. Individual therapy is the cornerstone of learning to manage BPD symptoms because they can be safely experienced in this private and controlled atmosphere. It isn't that the symptoms necessarily disappear, but that their power dissipates. Group therapy is the venue to explore belonging and gaining the support of peers who also are struggling. It is a place to learn about relationships and to practice putting language to feelings and needs.

Fortunately I was treated by two medical professionals who made it clear that they cared about me unconditionally. My therapist was ready to challenge my thinking in an incredibly compassionate way. She created a very safe environment for me in therapy and, importantly, she repeatedly told me that I was safe. She did not judge me, and she had the patience of a saint. This was important, because I am intensely self-critical. It wasn't easy to learn the best ways to help me because I had layers of secrets upon secrets. I had many different faces and roles that I thought I needed to use to relate to her. I played games involving emotional push and pull, and I lied so often that I lost track of my lies. We spent a lot of time figuring out my chosen behaviors and developing the preventive strategies to use in the next situation. This took a long time because I didn't understand honesty; I didn't understand how words translated into actions; and I didn't understand that I was trying to develop a relationship with myself and find out who I was.

The second medical professional was an excellent psychiatrist (also a skilled psychopharmacologist) who figured out the right medicines to make my treatment and healing more effective. Other medications that I was taking had to be considered; also my body, at age 45, was going through perimenopause, which made the puzzle more difficult. I was not always a willing participant in the discussions, but she helped me work through noncompliance issues and problems with side effects.

● ● ●

Old behaviors of reaching for a quick fix to ease emotional distress began to be painstakingly replaced with skillful and healthy reactions or actions.

● ● ●

I don't mean to say that these two medical professionals were easy on me. I was required to honor my contracts, and of course it was not always smooth sailing as I was taught the relationship between choice and consequence. I wouldn't be here without their constant support, and in the world of a BPD person, constant support is critical.

The third factor is a tangible means to give structure to the chaotic and random ways in which people with BPD interact with their environment, other people, and themselves. For me, attending New York Presbyterian Hospital's day treatment program offered miracles. I was safe, and in the warmth of this safety I wasn't so afraid. Highly trained therapists and struggling peers understood me, even with my limited and fragmented ability to express how I was feeling or what I was thinking. Gradually my life really began to change in that environment. There I was taught dialectical behavior therapy (DBT) skills. I was taught ways to focus my mind, and I learned to accept that feelings just are and can be tolerated—the positive as well as the negative ones—for there can be a lot of fear and mistrust about feeling good for a person with BPD. I learned how to recognize my escalating levels of distrust and was shown specific skills to use to help me cope and not act impulsively. I learned how to interact with people and to discover my triggers and sensitivities, and I acquired skills to help me face them. In group therapy practice, and with the help of peers, the words came more easily and were not so frightening for me to hear. Old behaviors of reaching for a quick fix to ease emotional distress began to be painstakingly replaced with skillful and healthy reactions or actions. Learning to relate to people, learning to talk, and learning the DBT skills takes practice, practice, and more practice. It isn't easy, but for me it has been well worth the effort! I would even venture to say that for anyone with BPD, it is well worth the effort.

● ● ●

There is nothing that can penetrate so deeply as having someone believe in your worth and your ability to get better. I can't stress enough the importance of family involvement. It is critical. I wouldn't be anywhere, maybe not even be here today, without the unconditional love and support of my family.

● ● ●

The fourth and final factor is the love and support of a spouse or life partner, a father or mother, a brother or sister. There is nothing that can penetrate so deeply as having someone with belief in your worth and in your ability to improve and get better. I can't stress enough the importance of family involvement. It is critical. I wouldn't be anywhere, maybe not even be here today, without the unconditional love and support of my family. They believed in me. They believed that I was capable of change, and they never stopped believing. My husband attended every kind of therapy session imaginable, learning skills to help me in times of distress, learning skills to help him when my emotional roller coaster became unbearable, reading articles and learning as much as he could. This was not a happy time for him, but he never gave up on me or on our relationship. In his not giving up, I learned the need to keep trying to learn to live with BPD.

Now, after several years, I have learned that I can safely feel both happy and sad. Do I still get emotional? Yes, but I can tolerate the feelings, both good and bad. Do I ever feel impulsive? Of course, but now I think before I act. Am I still deeply sensitive? Yes, but I am not afraid of that sensitivity any longer, and I understand when to reach out for help. Do I find myself ever starting to "split"? Unfortunately, the answer is yes, but not very often. I have learned how to safely interrupt the process and am continuing to learn how to express what is on the inside. I like interacting with the world, learning who I am, and feeling more at peace. What could be more important than that?

I continue to use learned skills every day of my life. I carry a much-loved index card in my purse for quick reference, and I have a crisis card to be used whenever I find myself not thinking clearly and feeling panicky. Learning new ways to cope and to interact with the world, unfortunately, will not change a person's memories or sensitivities. Triggers live around every corner, as my therapist says, and a person needs to be able to face them without falling apart or, in my case, "splitting." I carry a journal to write a kind word to myself on difficult days or to put language to distressing and confusing feelings, which at times can still be difficult for me. I know that life will deal me both good and bad, but I am confident that I can safely deal with both.

In the past few years I have returned to work full time, completed a master's degree in liberal studies and psychology, and begun to teach DBT and life-coping skills to those struggling with a mental illness and their families. I am in a unique position to help and teach others. I understand the complexities of feeling confused, feeling inadequate in using words, but desperately wanting to reach out. I know and understand what helps, and so I can teach skills for living through real-life examples and through offering skillful ways to handle difficult situations. As we work on ways to live in the moment and reduce distress, talk, role-play, and support each other's skillful strides, I feel thrilled and enriched to share what I have learned. As I say to myself every day: Take BPD by the hand. Don't be afraid!

References

Capote T: Breakfast at Tiffany's: A Short Novel and Three Stories. New York, Random House, 1958

Kernberg PF, Weiner AS, Bardenstein KK: Personality Disorders in Children and Adolescents. New York, Basic Books, 2000

Yeomans FE, Clarkin JF, Kernberg OF: A Primer of Transference-Focused Psychotherapy for the Borderline Patient. Northvale, NJ, Jason Aronson, 2002

• 7 •

Family Perspectives on Borderline Personality Disorder

Dixianne Penney, Dr.P.H.
Patricia Woodward, M.A.T.

A first encounter with borderline personality disorder (BPD) is likely to leave one reeling: a call from the emergency room or a counselor at school or college, or a knock on one's bedroom door at night with a cry for help. As emotions and actions can overwhelm and become overwhelming, family members and friends alike can spin off into their own mini-crises. They ask questions like "Why didn't we know?"; "What could we have done?"; "Why is this happening now?"; and "Where do we go from here?" Often family members will have opposing reactions, ranging from denying the seriousness of the situation to taking empathetic and sympathetic stances. But for the person whose life is falling apart, the last thing that is needed is for the people he or she loves and depends on to start falling apart.

Most parents encounter the term *BPD* for the first time when their child is diagnosed with the disorder. They might run to look up the diagnosis in the American Psychiatric Association's (2000) *Diagnostic and Statistical Manual of Mental Disorders,* 4th Edition, Text Revision, if they are familiar with that publication, but many parents do not even know that a psychiatric classification system called DSM-IV-TR exists. Most of us come by information and help the hard way.

● ● ●

It is our hope that effective treatments for
BPD will continue to be developed and that
affected individuals and their clinicians will
undertake treatment knowing that there can
be reasonable outcomes.

● ● ●

The two accounts that follow—about a young woman named Jesse and a father and his daughter—are stories of young adults with BPD told from the viewpoint of family members and friends. Although this chapter reflects the perspective of families with a young member diagnosed with BPD, we do not mean to minimize the gravity of BPD in adults. It is our hope that effective treatments for BPD will continue to be developed and made fully available for people of *all* ages, that the general public will be more knowledgeable about the disorder, and that affected individuals and their clinicians will undertake treatment knowing that there can be reasonable outcomes.

Getting the News: Dealing With the Diagnosis

Some 15 years ago, when talking with parents and educators about their first encounter with BPD, we heard one phrase repeated so often it became a refrain: "I had no idea what it was all about—If only we had known." When they shared the news with friends and other family members, the response heard most often by family members was, "What's that? Never heard of it." People's reaction to the diagnosis was one of bewilderment: "Borderline? Is that because it borders on schizophrenia?" In teachers' rooms the response sometimes was, "Don't give me that kind of nonsense. The kid's oversensitive. Just needs to pull herself together." Teachers are in the best position to recognize behaviors that might warrant adult intervention and support, yet their training offers them minimal exposure to the potential effects of developmental problems on students' behavior. And there is the prevailing myth that teenagers are, at best, a volatile group of people who will outgrow troubling behaviors.

There has been some progress in the development of general awareness about BPD. Today more people tell us that when they talk about BPD they get responses like "Yes, I've heard of that"; and "There have been some really good documentaries on mental health and depression on TV"; or "I've heard about BPD, but what is it really?" They might note that they have an acquaintance or family member who has or might have the disorder, but

"No one really talks about it, you know. It's as though it's some sort of secret."

Speaking out about a personal experience with mental illness takes courage, not only because of the response one might encounter, but because it means dredging up many past memories. These two stories from parents of young women diagnosed with BPD—one from a mother and one about a father—are presented to illustrate the reality of BPD for the affected families.

A Mother's Experience: From the Inside

"Mommy, I feel sad." I first heard those words when Jesse was 3 years old and in nursery school. In retrospect, I realize my daughter knew before anyone else that she was different. She had friends among the gentle children but wanted desperately to be accepted by the 3-year-old "in-group." When I spoke to her teachers, they said she was just shy, and as one of the youngest in her class she probably was not yet able to keep up. "She'll grow out of it," they assured me.

● ● ●

"Our friends' children were becoming young adults without too many ups and downs and within acceptable timetables. Our nieces and nephews were all excelling at everything they did. What could we say when someone asked, 'How's Jesse?'"

● ● ●

And so the years went by. Jesse grew into a beautiful, willowy young woman. As her nursery school teachers had predicted, she was a high achiever, a talented painter. She was well respected by her teachers and always had a few close friends. Nonetheless, she still saw herself as an outsider. As Jesse's description of her sad feelings grew more sophisticated, she asked if I thought she would ever belong. She said she felt as if everyone else knew what was going on, what was happening, how to act, but that she felt "clueless." This was hard for me to comprehend. She appeared so poised, so in charge of her life.

Although Jesse did not receive the diagnosis until she was in her early 20s, some symptoms of borderline personality disorder had already appeared. When she was diagnosed with borderline personality disorder, as awful as it seemed, it was a relief because finally we had some kind of explanation for symptoms we could not understand.

Jesse had always been a very slender child (just like her father, I told myself). During her teen years, she fooled both her pediatrician and me into believing that she was simply continuing her slender predisposition, because she always managed to stay just at the edge of low-normal weight. Nonetheless, she had acquired many manifestations of an eating disorder: bizarre eating habits, lying about her food intake, a completely distorted body image, and then, at about age 16, severe bulimia.

● ● ●

"Before we found a treatment program that embraced people with BPD and their families, we found that many clinicians wrote off persons with BPD as treatment resistant and their families as overinvolved."

● ● ●

Drug and alcohol abuse followed. Despite all this, Jesse continued to excel at school and in the creative arts. She was accepted at the prestigious college of her choice. I thought this ego boost would really help. Little did I know that this complex illness had already taken hold of her. I should have been alerted that something was terribly wrong when Jesse stopped painting soon after she arrived at college, but I was lulled into complacency by her insistence that she really needed more time for her studies. Shortly after the start of her sophomore year, her life and ours fell apart. Jesse withdrew from college and arrived home, weighing only 85 pounds at 5 feet 6 inches tall.

How isolated we all felt! Jesse was so ashamed and was afraid to ask for help. Although we knew something was dreadfully wrong, my husband and I were still in denial. How could it be that our beloved daughter was not only unable to cope with the usual activities of a bright and talented 18-year-old, but also was engaging in self-destructive behavior?

In terror for our child, we looked everywhere for an explanation. Finding none at the time, we looked inward. What had we done to cause this? Had the genes of her forebears produced these problems (we still weren't using the term *mental illness*), or was it the family environment during her childhood? We blamed ourselves. We also experienced for the first time a real (or was it perceived?) sense of stigma, not only from our friends but also from our own families. Our friends' children were becoming young adults without too many ups and downs and within acceptable timetables. Our nieces and nephews were all excelling at everything they did. What could we say when someone asked, "How's Jesse?"

Although we didn't know what was wrong with her, we knew we didn't want to tell anyone what was going on. We stopped sending greeting cards (where it seems one is expected to say at least something about the accomplishments of one's children). We started withdrawing from our social circle, and our relationships within our nuclear and extended families became strained. Life as we knew it had ended.

The stigma of this disease did not stop with friends and family. Before we found a treatment program that embraced people with the disorder and their families, we found that without listening to us or telling us exactly why they were not interested in treating our child, many clinicians wrote off persons with BPD as being treatment resistant and their families as being overinvolved. As a parent, I frequently felt that, at best, some therapists viewed me as someone whose IQ had just dropped 40 points because I had a child with BPD. Even more shocking and hurtful was the discovery that the major advocacy groups for persons with mental illness had little or no interest in BPD and in some instances even tried to stifle our family's cries for help and support.

We tried for years to get help for Jesse. Many therapists, several day programs, and five hospitalizations later, her reserves and hope for recovery were gone. One Sunday afternoon, we received the phone call from hell: "Your daughter has taken a massive overdose. She's at the emergency room. Please get here as soon as you can. She may not live." When we arrived, Jesse was in four-point restraint with tubes entering and exiting all over her body. I can scarcely remember the days that followed.

Someone had told me about a cognitive-behavioral therapy treatment, dialectical behavior therapy (DBT), developed by Dr. Marsha Linehan (1993a, 1993b), for the treatment of suicidal patients with BPD. It seemed a miracle that this treatment was available in our area and that there was a place for Jesse.

Once a week, multifamily group therapy was also offered as part of this program. My husband and I joined the group. Ideally, both the family and the person with BPD attend these sessions, where cognitive-behavioral skills based on DBT are taught to the group as a whole and where family members can practice communicating with one another in a safe setting. My husband and I were helped greatly by the group to grieve and let go of blame, to mourn and shed the burden of guilt, and to find relief from the additional agony of the stigma imposed by those who have not walked in our shoes.

At the time of Jesse's suicide attempt, I would not have thought it possible to have the strength to continue to hope for her recovery. Much of the teaching we have received during the multifamily group sessions has been from individuals with BPD who attended the group, most of whom were young women like Jesse. Their insights into what has been helpful to them, how to be supportive without smothering, when to take the initiative and not feel guilty, how to help our daughter fight back against stigma wherever it appears—even if it means standing up to a grandmother, in-law, or therapist—have made my husband and me able to take charge of our lives again. In doing so, we have become part of the team that has helped Jesse gain the courage and strength to take charge of her recovery.

It has been a long process and very hard work, but Jesse is eager and seems ready to reenter the workforce and complete her college degree, approaching each of her goals step by step. She has friends again and is looked upon as a leader among them. For a little while now we have had our daughter back, the Jesse we once knew and thought we might never see again.

A Father's Experience: From the Outside

This is a story of the effect of BPD on a family that I have witnessed as a friend. I have a very vivid memory of a hospital room. When I turn back from gazing out the window, I see seated on the very edge of the bed by the door a slip of a girl, just sitting there, head down, hands limply held together in her lap. Framed in the doorway stand three people: a mother, a father, and an older brother. They are transfixed standing there, frozen in time and place. The hospital is in a college town and the father has "professor" written all over him. A cursory glance shows that they are certainly well-put-together people, even at that time of crisis. A resident comes up behind them and as they slowly turn to leave, they seem to be a close family group, attentive to each other, and gentle in their manner and movement.

I happened on them a few hours later in the cafeteria. A divide was apparent. The son and mother were together, unmoving, passive, and quiet. The father was sitting a little apart, but attentive to the movements in the room, looking at the comings and goings. We exchanged glances, long enough so that when we met a few years later at another hospital we recognized each other. He had aged years, and was beyond desperation from grief and loss. His wife had left him and the son would not speak to him. The young girl had by then mothered two children, was going through a divorce, and would not allow the family to see the children. He feared for the young children, but futile attempts to obtain custody had driven the family members further apart. Despite consultations with many medical people, no one had been able to help the young girl, who had finally been diagnosed with BPD after several years of treatment for affective disorder, bipolar disorder, and substance abuse. At issue with his wife was abuse—sexual abuse in this case. The father's face—even his whole body—appeared contorted as he spoke of the accusations against him by his wife, who had done some reading on the causes of the disorder. The daughter herself had made no such accusation. The helplessness and confusion the family experienced at the time of the first hospitalization had continued for years. They had become lost in an emotional morass, in a confusion of apparently contradictory terms: overinvolvement and underinvolvement, enmeshment and dysfunction.

The father's personal despair finally drove him to seek long-term consultation with a family social worker who helped him develop a battery of self-caring skills. She invited him to attend her evening sessions with other parents at which issues of personality disorders were discussed. These weekly meetings over a 2-month period made a difference. He learned more about the characteristics and impact of personality disorders and was encouraged to revise his own role in the family and develop support relationships with other families.

●　●　●

The family had become lost in an emotional morass, in a confusion of apparently contradictory terms: overinvolvement and underinvolvement, enmeshment and dysfunction.

●　●　●

In some ways this father was unlucky that for many years lack of knowledge about BPD had so stressed his family that it had been irrevocably fractured by the overwhelming emotional and financial costs. But he was fortunate that he had finally found a clinician, a social worker motivated by personal interest who had acquired training in dealing with personality disorders and who had access to a progressive mental health infrastructure. The outcome was that the father acquired the communication skills to reestablish contact with his daughter. The change in his attitudes allowed his daughter to acknowledge her needs to him, and they are gradually mending their relationship.

Reflections on the Family Experience of BPD

BPD as Chronic Illness

When someone develops a chronic illness, the ripples are felt by all members of the family, the extended family, close friends, and employers. Everyone's behavior is affected. With some illnesses, it is possible to know how to behave because the illness is defined, the causes are known, the treatment is specified, and the course and outcome are certain. Chronic illness makes overwhelming demands even when the illness is known and understood. When the causes are not clear or specific, when diagnoses are moving targets, when treatment options are limited, and when outcomes are uncertain, the demands and burdens are that much greater.

● ● ●

Parents may feel that if they are responsible for causing the disorder, they can actually "cure" it. The therapist can help the family deal with these issues of guilt and blame.

● ● ●

When someone in the family receives a diagnosis of BPD, it is a life-changing event for that person and for that family. The family has to deal with the problems common to all chronic conditions, with the addition of factors and behaviors specific to BPD. The problems families face depend on whether the person with the diagnosis is living at home (no matter what age) or is away from home. If the person is under age 18 or if parents are responsible for the medical bills, then they also may have access to information on treatment. Being supportive is far more difficult if the ill relative is living away from home, has no access to information, and must secure emotional and financial support and negotiate issues of employment, insurance, and Supplemental Security Income.

Even if the ill relative is living at home, the questions remain: How do you know if he or she is receiving appropriate support for a disorder that can take several years to get under control? How do you measure progress when it is likely to be slow and even erratic? There is also the human tendency to avoid dealing with deeper issues when things are going well, even though these issues cannot be approached in times of crisis. Furthermore, it is usually not an option to discuss family issues with the relative's therapist. Therefore, an important issue for families is how to set up a communication channel where emotional and financial issues can be discussed and resolved. If the professionals involved view the family as dysfunctional and the parents as "causative" agents, it is doubly hard for the family to position itself in a supportive role.

Finding the Right Therapist

When an ill relative has problems beyond BPD, it is very hard even for the most loving and well-adjusted family to maintain integrity in family functioning. One thing, however, seems to be clear: if the individual with BPD has comorbid issues (e.g., depression, eating disorders, substance abuse, and alcohol abuse) and BPD is not addressed, the changes needed for the person to lead a stable life are harder to achieve. Of paramount importance is finding a trusted therapist who is willing to answer questions, explain the reasons for treatment, and help set treatment priorities, including emergency planning for crises. It is especially helpful if the therapist can work with the person with BPD and family members or significant others in dealing with boundary issues such as spending money, engaging in risky behaviors, and meeting agreed expectations at home and at work.

A therapist can also help the family deal with issues of guilt and blame. Often parents may feel that if they are responsible for causing the disorder, they can actually "cure" the problem. Because it seems that it takes a combination of factors and events to cause an individual to develop BPD, the corollary is that it will take a combination of therapy, support, and medications to enable someone to come to terms with the behaviors that result from the disorder. It takes a high level of training, skills, experience, and caring commitment to lead the person with BPD and the family—individually and at times jointly—through the incremental steps needed to bring about change.

What Families Need to Know About Hospital Treatment

Statistics show that approximately 10% of outpatients and 20% of psychiatric inpatients have BPD symptoms. Such a level of use of medical and clinical services surely indicates the seriousness of the disorder, not only for the person with BPD but also for the impact on health services. With reimbursement for mental health services in such a fluid state, consumers and families need to know the terms of their private and state medical insurance policies in detail. The fine print of these policies often proscribes services for mental illnesses, and the uncertainty about access to therapeutic services can be highly unsettling for the patient and family.

Family members also need to know the rules of the hospital or institution, as well as the rights of patients. The organization of treatment teams and level of staff training may vary greatly from one hospital to another. Institutional policies for dealing with families are not always family friendly, and without help from the hospital staff, it takes some doing to get used to the atmosphere and restrictions of a locked ward. In the volatile conditions that surround crisis-driven hospitalizations, the focus of staff is on the patient. It might seem to family members that they are suspect in their relationship with the person undergoing the crisis. New words enter one's vocabulary: *checks* (rounds made at regular intervals by hospital staff to check on safety of patients) and *sharps* (objects such as nail files or scissors, which may be used for self-harm) take on new meanings.

If you watch visitors on the hospital ward and in the cafeteria, it may appear to you that the people who are most at ease are those who have been through the routine many times before. They seem to know how to talk to the staff, when the doctors are available, and where the social workers' offices are. They have in fact learned the system. No doubt you will be able to learn it, too.

Dealing With the Stigma of Abuse

The stigmatizing aspects of BPD can permeate interactions with family members, with friends, and even with medical personnel and providers. The research literature and training materials for psychiatrists, psychologists, and social workers make references to the purported incidence of abuse—intentional or inadvertent—occurring among people diagnosed with BPD. If you happen to be consulting a therapist yourself to get help with the situation and the therapist comments that the child in question is acting like an abused child, this can have a powerful effect on your attitude toward family members and close friends. If you are a single parent and you know that you have not been abusive, then where did the abuse come from? If you are in an extended family, how do you then view the other people in the family who may have had access to your child? For parents, how do you then look at your own relationship? Did any abuse even occur? The issue for parents or concerned others is how the very likelihood of abuse and neglect affects their relationship with treatment teams or individual therapists. It is very hard to sit face to face with medical professionals and wonder what they are thinking about you or the family, just as it must be hard for clinicians to face people who may well have contributed to distress in their patient. You can understand the dilemma, but it is nevertheless very painful. Combined with the experience of dealing with the common reactions and the stigma of having a mentally ill person in your life, such attitudes of accusation add immeasurably to the isolation and burden of the family. In this new climate of suspicion, it is difficult to do what you must do: that is, to put your own feelings aside and focus on getting the help needed and providing the support the person with BPD requires.

Managing BPD in the Family Environment

Learning what kind of support a person needs means answering some tough questions. What are some of the conditions that are important to achieve in the family environment? What expectations or attitudes might family members need to work on or adapt? At times the person with BPD might seem well put together and very capable, so family members may have differing opinions as to what can or should be expected from her or him. For someone who at times feels very threatened and vulnerable, having family members be at odds is not useful, and so the family really needs to develop a unified approach; this may require working with a counselor to achieve a common approach and set priorities. Safety is usually the main priority, and the family should know whom to contact in case of emergency (intentional self-harm or abuse of medications, etc.) and should have such a plan in place. Setting limits and being able to state expectations clearly and honestly might be harder than one might think and involves understanding the difference between being supportive and enabling. It is far easier to explain expectations in calm times than to issue an ultimatum in the midst of an escalating argument.

All of us need to be involved in making decisions, and there is a learning curve entailed in being able to help someone under stress through a decision-making process in a collaborative and consistent manner. Although criticisms can be taken as challenges by the person with BPD, it is important for family members to learn not to respond in kind. All people have disagreements, but it is essential that we not escalate harsh feelings and that we stay in an attentive listening mode. If one is able to analyze the big problems and figure out ways to deal with them in smaller steps, then the family is less open to frustration and discouragement.

Making the Changes in Ourselves

Remaining optimistic and realistic takes determination and parallels what is being demanded of the person with BPD who, over extended periods of time, is being asked to make complex internal changes in monitoring emotions and patterns of feeling and thinking. Likewise, as family members we need to monitor our emotions and be aware of our own thinking patterns. It is very difficult to watch someone you care for experience intense psychological pain, and it often takes an act of faith to witness repeated setbacks. If we see behaviors as deliberately willful and hurtful, we will react to that. If we see the behaviors as reflecting a deficit in skills rather than a deliberate purpose, it provides more motivation to keep us alert to emotional cues and attentive to our own physical and mental well-being. We have learned that people with BPD lack self-soothing techniques. If we are to offer good modeling of emotional health, then we, the ones trying to be supportive, need to make sure we maintain good physical and emotional health. An old adage about being a parent cautions that you cannot look after someone else unless you are able to look after yourself. Parents and other family members may not think of themselves as "caretakers," in the mental health sense of the word, but that is in fact what we are. This means that we must learn to care for ourselves while striving to create a workable, comfortable family environment for our loved one with BPD.

● ● ●

If we are to offer good modeling of emotional health, then we, the ones trying to be supportive, need to make sure we maintain good physical and emotional health.

● ● ●

Finding Available Treatments for BPD

The stories in this chapter about Jesse ("A Mother's Experience: From the Inside") and the unnamed father ("A Father's Experience: From the Outside") began a number of years ago. Since then, major changes have occurred in service delivery, insurance coverage, research, and training of professionals with respect to BPD. Although services may be variable depending on where one lives, many centers offer a package of services beginning with the crisis when the young person receives the diagnosis of BPD. Parents are given a "road map" of what course of treatment will be offered. Rather than conducting family meetings with a judgmental atmosphere, families are supported and encouraged in specific ways to help their loved one through the crisis. The person with BPD might attend intensive counseling sessions, including ongoing training in DBT skills, often in a day treatment program. Some parents might find a hospital or institution that underwrites complementary parent support or psychoeducation programs, such as those described in this book, which offer information on the disorder, explain treatment options, teach communication skills, and help families develop support networks.

The future holds even more promise. Just as parents and professionals have joined together to advocate for the needs of individuals with schizophrenia and autism, a similar energy is being channeled into research on the causes of BPD and the means of treating the disorder more effectively. Some hospitals and institutions now serve as centers promoting model programs for research on and treatment of BPD. Perhaps one day it will be possible for all affected families to receive an accurate and timely diagnosis of BPD, an effective treatment program that meets individual needs, and support from family members and friends.

● ● ●

When families are given information and support to lessen their own traumatic experiences, they can become effective members of an extended treatment team.

● ● ●

As with most life events, there is a window of opportunity when someone is diagnosed with BPD. When Jesse came home from college, when the unnamed young mother was admitted to the hospital, those were the windows of time before the shock and reactions set in. It is at this time, the time of diagnosis, that judicious interventions of information and support can make an important difference to family members' handling the crisis and framing future moves. This is not a disorder people choose to have. When families are given information and support to lessen their own traumatic experiences, they can become effective members of an extended treatment team.

Living Your Own Life

In closing, there are a few additional thoughts we would like to share. We learned to hold on to hope, even though hope often hurts. When all seems lost, hope can be sustaining, and it may be the one thread your child is still able to grasp. We learned to search for programs and therapists that welcomed individuals with BPD and that appreciated family input and considered it important for both the short- and long-term well-being of the entire family. We were fortunate to find a support program that targets BPD and is designed for family members. We also learned to take care of ourselves. It is so easy to devote all your time, conversation, and energies to your sick child at the expense of the rest of life.

What gives relief will be different for each person. In spring, summer and fall, what helped was to find a few minutes each day to work in the garden; and in winter, it was helpful to take the time to arrange fresh flowers. Take time for yourself, time to be yourself! You have to know that you did the best you could at any one moment. You did not cause this illness any more than your child chose to have it.

References

American Psychiatric Association: Diagnostic and Statistical Manual of Mental Disorders, 4th Edition, Text Revision. Washington, DC, American Psychiatric Association, 2000

Linehan MM: Cognitive-Behavioral Treatment of Borderline Personality Disorder. New York, Guilford, 1993a

Linehan MM: Skills Training Manual for Treating Borderline Personality Disorder. New York, Guilford, 1993b

• 8 •

From Family Trauma to Family Support System

Harriet P. Lefley, Ph.D.

Across diagnostic categories, any serious mental illness is a traumatic event that brings confusion, grief, and altered lives both to patients and to their family members. There is now a substantial body of literature on the traumatic impact of psychiatric disorders such as schizophrenia and bipolar illness on families, including the burdens of caregiving. However, studies of borderline personality disorder (BPD) have focused largely on *etiology,* that is, on antecedent events and relationships that presumably gave rise to this particular diagnosis. There is very little information on how families experience the difficulties of living with BPD. In this chapter I therefore provide an overview of the literature on family burden in mental illness generally, most of it applicable to BPD. I also discuss research findings specific to families and BPD; these findings are used in the training of mental health professionals and may affect the subsequent attitudes of those professionals toward families. The implications of this training for relationships between families and professionals need to be explored. These relationships can be helpful or harmful to family members and may affect their ability to function as an adequate support system for their ill member.

Some actual experiences of families with BPD, ranging from living with the disorder to dealing with the mental health system, were derived from a family focus group session conducted in July 2002 (P.D. Hoffman, P. Woodward, D. Penney, et al., "Learning From Families," unpublished manuscript, 2003). This session compared events in the lives of families with BPD with those of families living with other major psychiatric disorders. Some family members have benefited from learning about evidence-based techniques that can be usefully applied in dealing with BPD behaviors and with their own reactions to the illness. At the conclusion of this chapter, I suggest ways in which families can live most supportively with their loved ones with BPD while maintaining the integrity of the family and the family members' right to live their own lives.

Families' Experiences With Mental Illness

The body of research on families' experience when one member has a mental illness suggests pervasive problems across diagnoses. There are objective burdens, such as the family's investments of time and energy in negotiating the mental health, social service, and often criminal justice systems; disruption of household routines; the mentally ill person's inability to fulfill expected role functions; economic dependence and financial costs of the illness; deprivation of needs of other family members such as siblings and children; curtailment of social activities; inability to fulfill personal plans; embarrassing situations and impaired relations with the outside world; and difficulties in finding adequate hospitalization or appropriate residential alternatives. There is also subjective burden: mourning the *premorbid personality;* grieving for what might have been; empathic suffering for the pain of a loved one; feeling stigma on one's own behalf as well as the patient's; and worrying about the future.

*Family members need to learn how to set limits,
to have appropriate expectations, and above all
to respect their own right to a decent life.*

● ● ●

Families may have to contend with a range of very difficult behaviors—projected rage, blaming, verbal or even physical abuse, denial of illness, and rejection of treatment. Above all, they must try to figure out limits, accountability, and expectations of appropriate behavior, typically without any professional help to guide them. Added to societal and situational stressors are the often censorious and distancing attitudes of mental health practitioners, the denial of information, and the lack of therapeutic resources both for persons with the illness and their families (Lefley 1996; Maurin and Boyd 1990; Schene et al. 1998).

Many of these problems obviously require larger solutions at the societal and mental health system levels. Their resolution calls for organization and advocacy, and the current organization of families of persons with BPD, the National Education Alliance for Borderline Personality Disorder (NEA-BPD), is a notable step in the right direction. But in the here and now, given the available resources, how is it possible to go from family trauma to family support system? Although psychotherapy is usually considered the appropriate treatment for trauma, the research on evidence-based family interventions has shown that families benefit most from psychoeducation (Dixon et al. 2001)—that is, basic information, support, and techniques on how to live with and manage the illness. Most current BPD family therapies begin with psychoeducation (e.g., Berkowitz and Gunderson 2002; Glick and Loraas 2001; Hoffman et al. 1999).

● ● ●

Most research articles continue to focus on childhood abuse as an antecedent—and presumably a trigger, if not a cause—of BPD. The presumption of childhood trauma is built into most therapeutic modalities for BPD.

● ● ●

All families of persons with BPD need to be educated about the illness: what is known and unknown about its presumed etiology, its symptoms, its biological and psychological *substrates,* and the medications that can be used in its treatment; and ways to recognize *prodromal* cues of *decompensation.* Family members need to learn the basics of good communication, behavior management, and problem-solving strategies. They need to understand that their own anger, guilt, anxiety, and frustration are normal responses, but that they can be controlled to avoid accelerating disturbed behaviors in a loved one. Family members need to learn how to set limits, to have appropriate expectations, and above all to respect their own right to a decent life. Families need to share their grief and their hopes with others, and they need support so that they themselves can become support systems for people they love. What can families expect from professionals? With BPD, the technology both for treating patients and for helping their families is much less tested than that in other disorders such as schizophrenia or bipolar disorder. There is also much less in the way of rigorous etiological research, and theories of family causation still abound.

Research on Families and BPD

Research on the history of BPD differs profoundly from studies of other psychiatric disorders. For example, current searches of the professional literature on families and schizophrenia are very unlikely to turn up anything on the *double bind,* or *schizophrenogenic* mothers, or any of the other family causation theories that were so frequently found in the literature of 25 or 30 years ago. Environmental effects generally refer to nongenetic sources of damage to the developing fetus, not to nurture. But in a recent literature search on families and BPD, at least 90% of the articles dealt exclusively with nurture. Most research articles continue to focus on childhood abuse as an antecedent—and presumably a trigger, if not a cause—of BPD. The presumption of childhood trauma is built into most therapeutic modalities for BPD.

Stigma of Childhood Abuse and Neglect

For most clinicians, childhood trauma is associated with poor parenting and neglect. The convictions of 30 or 40 years ago that bad parenting caused schizophrenia and other major mental disorders led to considerable agony and frustration for families (McFarlane and Beels 1983; Terkelsen 1982). Given this damaging history, it seems necessary to search very carefully for explanations of the origins of BPD. Achieving clarity on etiological factors is extremely important for building appropriate treatment models; for fostering interrelations of families, consumers, and professionals; and for alleviating patients' anger and families' confusion and guilt. The ultimate goal, of course, is long-range prevention.

Sexual abuse is considered one of the strongest antecedents of BPD. However, two obvious facts stand out in the research literature. First, the majority of people who report abuse of all kinds—verbal, physical, or sexual—are emotionally scarred by the experience, but they do not develop serious psychiatric disorders of the magnitude of BPD. Sexual abuse in childhood is more commonly associated with adult depression. A large study comparing patients with BPD and those with other *Axis II* personality disorders found that BPD patients were significantly more likely to report verbal, emotional, and physical abuse by parental caretakers, but not sexual abuse (Zanarini et al. 2000). When sexual abuse occurs it is often inflicted by someone known to the patient, but rarely by the biological parents. When parents are recollected negatively, it is more likely to be a complaint of insufficient concern—that they were not vigilant enough to protect the patient from the offender.

Alternative Explanatory Models

Although in this chapter I focus on what the family can currently do, a discussion of potential alternative interpretations can be instrumental in alleviating parental guilt and in shaping therapeutic endeavors. Most current psychiatric textbooks and the treatment guidelines of the American Psychiatric Association (2001) acknowledge an inherited predisposition for BPD. Yet the research literature continues to emphasize a history of childhood abuse, neglect, and abandonment, with the majority of studies based on *retrospective self-report.* The immediate interpretation is that parents of offspring who develop BPD actually do inflict more abuse than other parents. Moreover, this abuse is so serious and unavoidable that it leads to dissociation as a coping mechanism, hypersensitivity to stress, and an inability to relate meaningfully to other human beings.

● ● ●

It is difficult to determine whether the parents were actually uncaring, or whether the person with BPD was biologically unable to form the usual bond with a caregiver.

● ● ●

But there are many other possible interpretations. The data may mean that the person predisposed to develop BPD is exceptionally sensitive to the demands and punishments of ordinary child-rearing environments, which results in overwhelming memories of having been abused. It can also mean that the person with this predisposition is a difficult, hypersensitive child who is not as easy to live with as other children—who drains and frustrates parents who then let out their anger on the difficult child. So when studies are done years later, the adult with BPD remembers an undue amount of childhood abuse. And indeed in some cases these memories may be valid.

Chess and Thomas (1997) described innate differences in temperament among children, who from birth seem to fall into three categories: easy, difficult, and slow to warm up. Difficult children may be hypersensitive, with different biological wiring from their siblings, so there may be frequent power struggles between their needs and the parents' need for order and discipline. Bleiberg (2002) described children at risk of developing a borderline or narcissistic personality disorder as being overwhelmingly demanding and self-centered and having uncanny sensitivity and reactivity, as well as a capacity to manipulate others.

Self-report studies may indicate that persons with BPD feel inadequate bonding to the persons who reared them. For example, one study found that insecure, anxious, or ambiguous attachment and a perception of relative lack of caring from one's own mother were uniquely associated with borderline features, beyond what could be accounted for by childhood adversity experiences (Nickell et al. 2002). It is difficult to determine whether the parents were actually uncaring, or whether the person with BPD was biologically unable to form the usual bond with a caregiver. Young and Gunderson (1995) found that adolescents with BPD viewed themselves as significantly more alienated from their families than did adolescents with other personality disorders, perceptions that were at variance with those of their parents. Bailey and Shriver (1999) stated that there are relevant alternative explanations for the association between childhood sexual abuse and BPD. In a survey of psychologists, they found that relative to patients with other personality disorders or other patients seeking psychological help, people with BPD were rated as especially likely to misinterpret or misremember social interactions. They were also considered likely to have voluntarily entered destructive sexual relationships, perhaps even at a young age. There is a well-established dynamic of a search for love and protection leading to inappropriate sexual relationships, unfulfillable expectations, and feelings of betrayal. These memories may well lead to genuine perceptions of having been sexually exploited and abused.

Avoiding Blaming in the Search for Cause

One of the great dangers in this kind of explanatory model is that of blaming the victim. Like most disorders, BPD is highly heterogeneous in level, intensity, and the basic personality of the person with the disorder. Although *affect dysregulation* and relationship difficulties and inconsistency seem to be prevalent in most cases, not all people with BPD are self-destructive or manipulative. In fact, it should be assumed that many recollections of sexual abuse may be valid and that such incidents were not situationally brought on by the carelessness or affectional needs of the victim.

As in all mental illness, clinicians have to be very careful about causal attributions, negotiating between the dangerous shoals of blaming the family and blaming the patient. Of all the explanatory models offered for this skewed history of abuse, the most parsimonious and most logical explanation may well be the one most frequently offered by sympathetic therapists and distraught parents. That is, the person biologically predisposed to develop BPD is hypersensitive to and more intensely experiences the normal slights, criticisms, and punishments endured by most children in the process of growing up. And if parents are raising an exceptionally difficult child, these criticisms and punishments are likely to be frequent and to generate tension in family dynamics—and later to be recalled as abusive.

Importance of Searching for Cause

If families are to be involved as a support system, there must be some plausible answers to their questions and their bewilderment. Some families will deny that anything exceptional happened in rearing the person with BPD. A few will say that their child rearing was benign, but that they later learned of sexual abuse by a hired caregiver or someone outside the family. Some will admit to having administered harsh punishments. But most simply cannot understand why there is a presumption of abuse so unbearable that it has led to such pathological behavior and misery in one of their children. The existing body of theory on the psychosocial antecedents of BPD presupposes a rearing history that many families simply do not recognize as damaging enough to lead to manipulation, fears of abandonment, self-mutilation, or attempted suicide. And they do not understand why their other children turned out so differently.

Moreover, there is apparent inconsistency in the findings that BPD is associated *both* with the presence of overly abusive parents *and* with no parents—with their actual loss through death, illness, or abandonment. Granted, children raised in foster homes are more likely to have experienced abuse, including sexual abuse, in these environments. However, these are not the caregivers who are willing to undergo family therapy or to belong to advocacy organizations to help their loved ones. These concerned and cooperative parents inevitably fluctuate between bewilderment, anger, and a guilt that is only dimly understood. There must be some explanation of their very different perception of events.

A second reason it is important to look for causality is that etiological theories inform and shape the treatment premises of individual psychotherapy and family interventions. Regardless of caveats in their training, theories of defective parenting inevitably affect the attributions and attitudes of the mental health professionals who offer these interventions.

Causal Attributions, Clinical Training, and Family–Professional Relationships

In a family therapy textbook, a chapter on BPD states that "*hard* data are accumulating that there are disturbed biological substrates in the patient....There is *suggestive* evidence that disturbed biology in combination with a disturbed "bad fit" family is etiologic in borderline personality disorder." (Glick and Loraas 2001, p. 141, emphasis in original). However, as in most of the literature, the research overview in this chapter has sections titled "Evidence of Family Pathology"; "Physical and Sexual Abuse"; "Neglect and Overprotection" and "Parental Pathology" (Glick and Loraas 2001, pp. 137–140). The authors make a sincere effort to be objective and state that "no evidence exists that pathologic family relationships *alone* can cause borderline personality disorder" (p. 141). Yet students are informed that "many borderline patients have been found to have **impulsive** and chaotic family environments in which physical and sexual abuse occur" (p. 138) and that "borderline patients described their parents as less caring than other parents" (p. 139). As in most texts, this otherwise valuable chapter reports the findings without exploring alternative explanations.

● ● ●

There are major barriers to working success-
fully with families when clinicians are con-
vinced that the cause lies in defective child
rearing.

● ● ●

Certainly the patients' own perceptions, regardless of objective fact, have to be acknowledged in therapeutic work. But with so much of the literature focusing on childhood abuse and neglect, many students reading this textual material are bound to develop a mindset that views families as sick and etiologically culpable. There are major barriers to working successfully with families when clinicians are convinced that the cause lies in defective child rearing. This premise, this theoretical model of the etiology of a whole range of serious mental illnesses, has led to therapeutic interventions that at best have failed to alleviate symptoms and at worst have damaged families and family-patient relationships. Mc-Farlane and Beels (1983) pointed out the implicit double bind in the dual messages conveyed to families by basically disapproving clinicians. "If one accepts that double-bind interactions can create distorted, even irrational communication, then many therapeutic situations can be seen as pathogenic. For example, covert blame of the family by professionals is often combined with overt attempts to help them, while the contradiction is denied" (p. 316).

The older family systems models have been unsuccessful with schizophrenia and bipolar disorder, and these models have been unsuccessful with BPD as well. Yet there is no doubt that any mental illness—certainly including BPD—has a profoundly shattering effect on the family system. Systemic interventions that work to strengthen equitable relationships and to reduce overinvolvement and the burden of guilt are to be welcomed. But clinicians need to avoid systemic interventions that view the symptoms primarily as a response to what goes on in the family, or as functional for maintaining a spurious homeostasis in the family economy. Furthermore, *enmeshment,* overinvolvement, *triangulation,* arguing, blaming, and other tortured dynamics of family systems can emerge as typical responses when incomprehensible stressors make people feel helpless and confused. These are maladaptive but normative responses. They have little or nothing to do with what causes the illness, but they may very well influence its severity and course.

Families' Experiences With Different Disorders

Although there are many common experiences across diagnostic conditions, there do seem to be differences between the major psychotic disorders and BPD. The focus group forum conducted in July 2002 ("Learning From Families," unpublished, 2003) highlighted commonalities and differences among families of people with BPD, schizophrenia, and the major affective disorders (primarily bipolar disorder). The common concerns voiced by families across diagnoses (Table 8–1) included handling patients' denial and rejection of treatment and their behavioral immaturity; assessing responsibilities to patient's siblings; dealing with patients' conflict with siblings and others in the household; and worrying about *prognosis* and the patient's future. There were concerns about preferred housing arrangements (i.e., living with the patient in the same household or elsewhere) and an appreciation of the value of support groups for families and of the advocacy roles they might assume.

● ● ●

Parents of children with BPD recalled that they had few rewards and many torments throughout the life cycle and did not really expect things to get much better.

● ● ●

Themes generated in discussion of the mental health system included feeling traumatized by the system; misdiagnosis and minimization of symp-

Table 8–1.	Concerns shared by families of people with major psychiatric disorders (including borderline personality disorder)

- Handling the family member's denial of the illness and rejection of treatment
- Handling behavioral immaturity
- Dealing with conflicts in the household
- Figuring out housing arrangements (i.e., living with the relative in the same household or elsewhere)
- Experiencing difficulty interacting with the mental health system
- Worrying about prognosis and the relative's future

Source. Hoffman PD, Woodward P, Penney D, et al: "Learning From Families," unpublished manuscript, 2003.

toms; uncertain or multiple diagnoses, especially for BPD; inappropriate medications or difficulty *titrating* the dosage levels; and confidentiality barriers. Families felt that multiple hospitalizations yielded little in the way of long-term benefit, and for some, incarceration of the family member with BPD seemed to be the only way to obtain treatment. Many families complained of receiving mixed or inconsistent messages from professionals. And as an interesting highlight on disciplinary training, many families agreed with the statement of one of the participants: "Psychiatrists welcome families. Therapists reject families." Most of the families of BPD patients knew about dialectical behavior therapy (DBT; Linehan 1993a, 1993b). They found the concept of the invalidating environment most beneficial, because it finally gave them a way of modifying their own behavior.

In the comparison of families' experiences with diagnosticians (Table 8–2), BPD seems more likely than other disorders to have been accompanied by multiple diagnoses or actual *comorbidity* (e.g., major depression or bipolar disorder, posttraumatic stress disorder, or eating disorders). These families have had to deal with a large array of disturbed behaviors. Many parents of people with schizophrenia or bipolar disorder remember the relationship with their children as having been rewarding when the children were in their premorbid states. However, parents of people with BPD often have contended with cognitive irrationality and mood swings in their child since childhood or early adolescence. Histories of self-mutilation and suicide attempts were more consistently symptomatic of BPD. Recollections suggested that parents of children with BPD had few rewards and many torments throughout the life cycle and did not really expect things to get much better. What they seemed to get from group interaction was understanding and confirmation rather than any easy answers.

Table 8–2. Additional concerns shared by families of people with borderline personality disorder

- Dealing with multiple diagnoses or comorbid disorders (e.g., major depression, posttraumatic stress disorder, substance abuse, or eating disorders)
- Dealing with a wide array of disturbed behaviors, including antisocial behavior and verbal abuse
- Dealing with irrationality and mood swings since the relative's childhood or adolescence
- Witnessing the relative's repeated self-mutilation and suicidal threats or attempts
- Obtaining comfort from group encounters but no easy answers

Source. Hoffman PD, Woodward P, Penney D, et al: "Learning From Families," unpublished manuscript, 2003.

Research by Hooley and Hoffman (1999) on expressed emotion also suggests differences between the responses of people with schizophrenia and bipolar disorder and those of people with BPD. High expressed emotion in a family member is essentially defined as hostile criticism toward or emotional overinvolvement with the patient. People with schizophrenia and bipolar disorder have a greater tendency to relapse under these conditions, whereas people with BPD seem to respond positively to emotional overinvolvement. The researchers suggested that heightened concern and overprotectiveness may be perceived as a kind of validation by people with BPD.

It is known that people with BPD seem to be more functional than people with psychotic disorders. People with BPD do not have obvious delusions or hallucinations, and they do not shut down completely like people with clinical depression. The negative symptoms of withdrawal, apathy, and *anhedonia* do not usually apply. Although it is true that in schizophrenia, negative symptoms are more burdensome to families than positive ones, this is because *florid* psychotic features are episodic and are usually controlled by medication. Withdrawn behaviors may be burdensome, but they are easier to live with than the emotional *lability* and demanding behaviors of BPD. Affect in BPD also differs from the intense anguish of depressive states. Loved ones may find it easier to forgive the pain caused by suicidal gestures if such acts seem to arise from a deep, unbearable depression. Because of their lability and manipulative histories, people with BPD evoke attributions of deficits in character rather than brain chemistry. It is very hard for families to see them as sick when they are so functional in other ways and so disturbingly inconsistent in their interactions with other people. Yet families of people with BPD, like the others, will often excuse outrageous behaviors by ascribing such behaviors to the illness. It is this see-sawing between accountability and nonaccountability, this confusion about the best way to behave, and of course the unpredictable cycling of behavior that makes life so difficult for families.

Helping the Family Become a Support System

With any mental illness, to alleviate trauma and become a viable support system, family members must learn a new set of three Rs: *recognizing, resisting,* and *reconstructing.* The first phase is learning to recognize behaviors that are purposeful and those that seem to be inherent in the illness and hard to control. The second phase is resisting being drawn into the vortex of dysregulation and irrationality. It means knowing how to set limits that define your own needs in relation to those of your loved one. It means knowing when to simply observe and when to take action either on your own behalf or on behalf of the loved one. This may be the hardest part of the learning process, but it also may be the most necessary factor for arriving at the third phase. This last phase involves reconstructing a meaningful relationship with a loved one who has seemed to be incapable of relating in meaningful ways.

Recognizing

Family members must first recognize that although they may be harassed, accused, or threatened, it is their relatives with BPD who feel like victims: people who have BPD feel victimized by others' inability to understand them. They feel that they live in a world in which those who claim to love them do not recognize and refuse to honor their pressing needs. Yet they themselves do not recognize the effects of their behavior on others—the embarrassing and difficult situations they create for their families.

● ● ●

Families that have a member with BPD inhabit a world of distorted mirrors. Communication is difficult because of vastly different perceptions, and families that contest these perceptions create what has been aptly called the invalidating environment.

● ● ●

Patients and families clearly see things differently. A study of the impact of BPD on patients and families found that patients were burdened by their symptoms, whereas families were burdened by their adult children's antisocial behavior. The findings showed that the majority of the patients, almost two-thirds, knew and regretted that their families were burdened by financial strain due to their increased dependency and inability to obtain jobs. Yet they were generally unaware of the awkward situations their behavior created for their families (Schulz et al. 1985).

Families that have a member with BPD inhabit a world of distorted mirrors. Communication is difficult because of vastly different perceptions, and families that contest these perceptions create what has been aptly called the invalidating environment (Linehan 1993a, 1993b). As noted above (see "Families' Experiences With Different Diagnostic Disorders"), families at the July 2002 forum found this concept exceptionally valuable. They seemed to recognize that *invalidation* trivializes or minimizes the other's perceptions and that they could learn to control this reaction on their part.

Resisting

It must be exceptionally hard to stay calm and avoid conflict when a family member is acting out outrageously. These are the situations in which recognition of the substrates of BPD—the affect dysregulation; the fluctuating, swirling emotionality—can lead to an understanding of why family members need to resist being drawn into its currents. Family members' anger, criticism, and rejection can heighten the fragmentation of the patient's uncontrollable world. Therefore families need to be taught that although these are not unnatural responses to difficult behaviors, they are hard on the nervous systems of people with hypersensitivity to these types of verbal and attitudinal stimuli and with a totally different perception of reality.

BPD can also entail emotional outrage when families refuse to yield to inappropriate demands. The task for families is to be able to acknowledge the feelings without showing hostile defensiveness and, unless they can be negotiated, without yielding to difficult demands. Keeping one's cool—maintaining boundaries without rejection—is something professionals learn to do, often despite extreme provocation. Family members can also learn to achieve this kind of composure. Such behavior is self-reinforcing because it tends to be effective in defusing emotional storms.

Professionals and Resistance

In treating BPD, professionals need to learn not only resistance techniques, but also how to correctly assess their patients' disclosures about their relations with their families. A study of adult psychiatric patients found that that the patients described parents at a more primitive conceptual level and expressed significantly more negativity and ambivalence than did psychiatrically healthy control subjects. In contrast to adults with no psychiatric diagnosis, who were able to evaluate their parents objectively, those with psychiatric disorders focused "mainly on gratification or frustration provided to the subject by the parent, with little recognition of the parents as complex individuals (with their own needs)" (Bornstein and O'Neill 1992, p. 481). Gunderson and Lyoo (1997) reported similar negativity toward parents in patients with BPD, despite the normative family relations described by their parents. According to psychiatrist Mary Seeman (1988), these adverse perceptions apply to psychotherapists as well: "The more attached a patient is to relatives or therapists, the more viciously the patient may attack them for disappointing him or her by not being perfect" (p. 98).

This behavior is easily recognized in persons with BPD. Their perceptions of the failings of the major protectors—of the inability of the once all-powerful parents to make life better—can generate terror and rage in their own fragile personalities with crumbling ego boundaries. This existential betrayal appears consistently among all kinds of adults who function at an immature level, and it may be prominent in major mental illness.

Reconstructing the Relationship

How then do both family members and professionals develop an equitable relationship with a person with BPD—a relationship that respects the person's otherness while understanding and resisting being drawn into his or her irrationality? It is beyond the scope of this chapter to give more than a few cursory examples. Many more comprehensive examples may be found in the family guidelines developed by Gunderson and Berkowitz (2002) for the New England Personality Disorder Association (see also Berkowitz and Gunderson 2002). The DBT–family skills training of Hoffman et al. (1999) has led to an offshoot, the Family CONNECTIONS program. This 12-week program, taught by trained family members, emphasizes nonjudgmental acceptance of persons with BPD as they are. Families learn that when they stop fighting the reality of BPD they can begin to focus more on positive aspects and things they can actually change.

What are some specific examples of what families can do? One useful tool is learning ways of dealing with verbal abuse. Abusive language should not be answered in kind but defused with a calm response. Family members should be able to recognize the feelings underlying an unjust accusation such as "You're never there for me!" to a mother or spouse of enduring forbearance. The statement itself may reflect fear of abandonment rather than an actual conviction of the other's indifference. The family member has to resist angrily protesting "I've always been there for you!"—a reply that gives legitimacy to the words. Calmly reaffirming "I'll always be there for you" ignores the accusation but is directly responsive to the underlying fear. Then the family member can reaffirm her own personhood and equity in the relationship by saying, "But I want you to be there for me, too, because we care about and need each other."

The DBT–Family Skills Training Model

Establishing equity is extremely important in stabilizing family relationships. The DBT–family skills training model developed by Hoffman et al. (1999) combines education about BPD with training in how to establish a mutually validating environment. In this short-term intervention, the family is taught to reinforce effective functioning in a consistent manner. At the same time, the patient is taught to reinforce effective parental interactions. The model is based on the premise that mutual reinforcement between patients and family members offers greater possibilities for change. This recognition of equity, of shared responsibility, is very important for implementing therapeutic change both intrapersonally and in enhanced family relationships. The mutual techniques enable participants to master situations and feelings that formerly seemed to spin out of control. The techniques may also reinforce feelings of family unity and support, with the potential for countering the fears of abandonment that are so ubiquitous in BPD.

● ● ●

With BPD, families may have to constantly reaffirm their commitment to stand by their ill family members and the need to understand that the complaints and accusations of the ill member are often generated by a desperate fear of abandonment.

● ● ●

In the skills training model of Hoffman et al. (1999), family members are taught to be less judgmental and less critical, to hear each other, and to interpret verbalizations in a benign way. In the focus group, however, the concept of validation was sometimes misconstrued as being placating rather than hearing and acknowledging another's perspective. I also saw something of what family therapist Ken Terkelsen (1982) called "the magical aspect of the wish to be blamed." Quite a few parents refuse to give up their cushion of guilt for having somehow brought on or exacerbated the illness. The magical aspect, of course, is thinking, "If I caused it, I can make it go away."

It is important for family members to accept the reality that the illness is not their fault and that they cannot cure the condition of their loved one. Certainly families can learn ways to improve the relationship. One way is by understanding that validation is not appeasement. Family members can learn that it is possible to reject a nonconsensual interpretation of events without being critical and judgmental. Family members can understand that the toxic kind of invalidation is that which disregards or trivializes others' perceptions and, most especially, minimizes their pain. Sometimes one person simply disagrees with another's viewpoint. It is easy enough to acknowledge that the other person sees things in a different way and then to search for things on which they do agree. An invalidating environment does not create the illness; rather, it reinforces the person's panic and anger at not being heard or understood. Although family members may find it difficult to understand ideas that do not correspond with their own reality, they can learn to accept another's perceptions at face value without criticism or rejection. If this becomes the modal behavior in the family, the member with BPD can begin to learn that rejection of a viewpoint or a behavior does not mean rejection of the person. Internalization of this recognition in the home would have a powerful effect on improving relationships with people in the outside world.

People with BPD must contend with a frightening and fragmented inner world. Their extremely difficult behaviors are maladaptive ways of coping with that world—an attempt to find security. A support system counters the fragmentation by providing form, structure, limits, and boundaries. Calmness, acceptance, and an avoidance of ambiguity and conflict are probably essential elements in any household that copes with mental illness. With BPD, families may have to constantly reaffirm their commitment to stand by their ill family members and the need to understand that the complaints and accusations of the ill member are often generated by a desperate fear of abandonment. Families also act therapeutically by appreciating their rights to satisfy their own needs and the needs of others in the household. By doing so, they reinforce the existential reality that the patient lives in a world in which the rights of other people must also be respected. This kind of support system offers the best basis for maintaining the integrity of the family system and for drawing secure boundaries around a chaotic inner world.

Finally, I want to strongly endorse what family members themselves said in the July 2002 focus group meeting. Becoming a support system involves more than acquiring knowledge alone. Families need their own support group for mutual sharing of experiences, for developing coping strategies, for learning about resource information, and for just experiencing the empathic understanding of others who have "been there." They need to become involved in advocacy for research and appropriate services. Learning and sharing and advocating become effective ways of helping not only one's own family, but also all those others who experience or live with BPD.

What Families Need to Know

Key Messages in This Chapter

- Families of people with BPD must deal with an array of objective and subjective burdens in coping with the illness, often without basic information or education about BPD or the help of professionals to guide them.
- One of the major hurdles for families seeking treatment for a relative with BPD is the lingering belief among mental health professionals that families are somehow responsible for the disorder.
- Despite recent evidence of a genetic predisposition to the development of BPD, much of the professional literature on BPD and families continues to focus on childhood trauma, abuse, and neglect as a trigger or cause of BPD.
- These assumptions about faulty child rearing learned by mental health professionals during their training can lead to treatment that is both unsuccessful *and* damaging to patient and family.
- Family members need concrete tools to help them deal with the dysregulated emotions and antisocial behavior of their relative with BPD. Families and patients can learn these skills through several programs based on the principles of dialectical behavior therapy (DBT).
- Families need to give up "the wish to be blamed" and accept the reality that just as they did not cause the condition of their loved one, they cannot cure it.
- Families can work to build a support system that *recognizes* the reality of their relative's BPD, *resists* becoming drawn into the emotional turmoil without rejecting her or him, and begins to *reconstruct* the rela-

tionship with their loved one. In the process, families need their own support system to share experiences, learn coping strategies, and gain comfort and encouragement from others who have "been there."

Key Words in This Chapter

affective   pertaining to one's emotional state.

anhedonia   a loss of interest in things that once brought pleasure.

Axis II   a classification in DSM-IV-TR (American Psychiatric Association 2000) that includes personality disorders such as borderline personality disorder.

comorbid   occurring together with another disease or condition.

decompensation   a failure of the defense mechanisms, leading to a relapse in symptoms.

double bind   a now-discredited theory of the causation of schizophrenia in which conflicting messages are given to children by parents.

dysregulation   the inability to regulate or control mood or impulses.

enmeshment   emotional overinvolvement in the relationship between two (or more) family members.

etiology   cause or presumed cause.

florid   fully expressed, as in psychiatric symptoms.

impulsivity   inability to resist performing some action that is harmful to oneself or others.

invalidation   a failure to legitimize the emotions, thoughts, and experiences of another.

lability   rapid fluctuation.

labile   unstable, changeable.

premorbid personality   the state of mental health before the onset of a disorder.

prodromal   before the onset of symptoms.

prognosis   prediction about the course of a condition or the chance for recovery.

retrospective self-report   a type of study design in which individuals with a given condition look backward in time to report on events in the past that may be associated with the condition.

schizophrenogenic   capable of causing schizophrenia.

substrate   the underlying layer or foundation.

titrating   determining the optimal level (of medication) to control symptoms.

triangulation   an alliance formed between a child and one parent (usually) that serves to isolate the other parent.

References

American Psychiatric Association: Diagnostic and Statistical Manual of Mental Disorders, 4th Edition, Text Revision. Washington, DC, American Psychiatric Association, 2000

American Psychiatric Association: Practice guideline for the treatment of patients with borderline personality disorder. Am J Psychiatry 158 (suppl):1–52, 2001

Bailey JM, Shriver A: Does childhood sexual abuse cause borderline personality disorder? J Sex Marital Ther 25:45–57, 1999

Berkowitz CB, Gunderson JG: Multifamily psychoeducational treatment of borderline personality disorder, in Multifamily Groups in the Treatment of Severe Psychiatric Disorders. Edited by McFarlane WR. New York, Guilford, 2002, pp 268–290

Bleiberg E: How to help children at risk of developing a borderline or narcissistic personality disorder. Brown University Child and Adolescent Behavior Letter 18(6):1–304, 2002

Bornstein RF, O'Neill RM: Parental perceptions and psychopathology. J Nerv Ment Dis 180:475–483, 1992

Chess S, Thomas A: Temperament: Theory and Practice. New York, Brunner/Mazel, 1997

Dixon L, McFarlane WR, Lefley H, et al: Evidence-based practice for services to families of people with psychiatric disabilities. Psychiatr Serv 52:903–910, 2001

Glick ID, Loraas EL: Family treatment of borderline personality disorder, in Family Therapy and Mental Health: Innovations in Theory and Practice. Edited by MacFarlane MM. New York, Haworth, 2001, pp 135–154

Gunderson JG, Berkowitz C: Family Guidelines: Multiple Family Group Program at McLean Hospital. Belmont, MA, New England Personality Disorder Association, 2002

Gunderson JG, Lyoo IK: Family problems and relationships for adults with borderline personality disorder. Harv Rev Psychiatry 4:272–278, 1997

Hoffman PD, Fruzzetti AE, Swenson R: Dialectical behavior therapy—family skills training. Fam Process 38:399–414, 1999

Hooley JM, Hoffman PD: Expressed emotion and clinical outcome in borderline personality disorder. Am J Psychiatry 156:1557–1562, 1999

Lefley HP: Family Caregiving in Mental Illness. Thousand Oaks, CA, Sage, 1996

Linehan MM: Cognitive-Behavioral Treatment of Borderline Personality Disorder. New York, Guilford, 1993a

Linehan MM: Skills Training Manual for Treating Borderline Personality Disorder. New York, Guilford, 1993b

Maurin JT, Boyd CB: Burden of mental illness on the family: a critical review. Arch Psychiatr Nurs 4:99–107, 1990

McFarlane WR, Beels CC: Family research in schizophrenia: a review and integration for clinicians, in Family Therapy in Schizophrenia. Edited by McFarlane WR. New York, Guilford, 1983, pp 311–323

Nickell AD, Waudby CJ, Trull TJ: Attachment, parental bonding, and borderline personality features in young adults. J Personal Disord 16:148–159, 2002

Schene AH, van Wijngaarden B, Koeter MW: Family caregiving in schizophrenia: domains and distress. Schizophr Bull 24:609–618, 1998

Schulz PM, Schulz SC, Hamer R, et al: The impact of borderline and schizotypal personality disorders on patients and their families. Hosp Community Psychiatry 36:879–881, 1985

Seeman MV: The family and schizophrenia. Humane Med 4:96–100, 1988

Terkelsen KG: The straight approach to a knotty problem: managing parental guilt about psychosis, in Questions and Answers in the Practice of Family Therapy, Vol. 2. Edited by Gurman AS. New York, Brunner/Mazel, 1982, pp 179–183

Young DW, Gunderson JG: Family images of borderline adolescents. Psychiatry 58:164–172, 1995

Zanarini MC, Frankenburg FR, Reich DB, et al: Biparental failure in the childhood experiences of borderline patients. J Personal Disord 14:264–273, 2000

• 9 •

Family Involvement in Treatment

Alan E. Fruzzetti, Ph.D.
Jennifer L. Boulanger, B.A.

The involvement of family in the treatment of serious psychiatric disorders experienced by other family members has been shown to be helpful both for the patient and for the family itself. The emerging data also support various types of family involvement in the treatment of borderline personality disorder (BPD), although studies to date are limited in number. The purpose of this chapter is to describe the different ways that family members can be involved in treatment and to review the available evidence supporting these approaches.

Unfortunately, many of the treatment programs described here are available only in limited geographic areas. If a program is not available locally, families might consider contacting the organizations or authors mentioned in this chapter for more information. Treatment providers may also contact the directors of these programs and request that training materials or course modules be made available. Our hope is that having consumers who are more knowledgeable will lead to the development and availability of programs that work.

Understanding Relevant Studies

It is important to clarify how health care and mental health care professionals evaluate the many different kinds of research. Consumers and professionals alike can easily be confused when proponents of one approach interpret evidence one way while proponents of another approach interpret evidence very differently.

For our purposes, controlled studies provide the most reliable evidence of a treatment's effectiveness. Other published reports, such as *case studies,* can be useful but do not constitute much evidence by themselves. The *randomized controlled trial* is the gold standard of scientific study. In a randomized controlled trial, one can be confident that the results are produced by the treatment being studied and not by some other unknown factor (or factors). In these studies, patients are randomly assigned to one of several different treatments before the outcome is evaluated. For this reason, special emphasis is placed on interventions that have been evaluated using this method.

Other types of controlled studies are also important and allow some confidence that the results are meaningful. Even uncontrolled studies are promising and suggest potentially useful approaches. However, the complete absence of research is problematic, and individuals with BPD and their families should be wary of treatments or programs that lack research evidence that they work.

There are effective ways that family members can become involved in the treatment of their loved one with BPD. These include 1) family involvement in treatment that is primarily designed to help the patient but is also focused on improving family relationships and family functioning in general; and 2) peer-led programs for family members designed to reduce stress and burden and to increase support.

● ● ●

The primary goal of family support or family education programs is to reduce the stress and burden of caring for a family member with a severe psychiatric disorder.

● ● ●

Family Involvement to Improve or Augment Patient Outcomes

Family members often want to know what they can do to maximize the recovery and minimize relapse for their loved one with BPD and related disorders. At least two broad types of programs are promising: family *psychoeducation* and certain types of *family therapy*. Most family psychoeducation programs are designed to supplement a patient's individual treatment (including psychotherapy and medications), and the primary goal is to improve outcome for the individual with BPD. These programs also may have the added benefit of reducing stress and improving support in families. Similarly, some forms of family therapy are designed specifically to supplement or augment individual treatment, often with good results. We first describe family psychoeducation programs in general and then psychoeducation programs for BPD more specifically.

● ● ●

Unlike conventional family therapy, which tends to assume dysfunction within the family, psychoeducation groups build on families' strength and resilience and do not blame family members for the patient's difficulties.

● ● ●

Family Education and Psychoeducation

Family psychoeducation was originally developed in the late 1970s for families with a member diagnosed with schizophrenia. Mental health professionals came to realize that family members played a significant role in the recovery of schizophrenic patients after an acute episode of illness and also that having a family member with a serious psychiatric disorder was stressful to the family as a whole. Individuals who improved the most were those in families fortunate enough to have access to accurate information about their specific disorder and a support system whereby they could learn from the trials and errors of other families facing similar challenges (McFarlane et al. 2003). Recognizing that most families did not have access to these kinds of resources, professionals began to offer structured psychoeducation groups in which family members could learn about their loved one's illness and how to respond to him or her more effectively.

Family psychoeducation groups vary in structure and format, but typically they are led by mental health professionals in treatment settings and are specific to a particular diagnosis or disorder (e.g., schizophrenia, bipolar disorder, or BPD). Unlike conventional family therapy, which tends to assume dysfunction within the family and focuses on solving family problems as a means to improve the individual's symptoms, psychoeducation groups build on families' strength and resilience and do not blame family members for the patient's difficulties. These groups provide illness-specific information and coping strategies aimed at improving patients' functioning and reducing caregiver burden.

William McFarlane built on the psychoeducation model by bringing several families together in a group format to learn from and support each other under the direction of a mental health professional. He also developed a new curriculum based on research findings showing that patients from families with a high level of negative *expressed emotion* were more likely to experience a relapse of psychiatric symptoms. Although these kinds of reactions can be understandable responses to the stresses of caring for a relative with severe mental illness, family psychoeducational interventions designed to change these patterns have been very helpful to patients and their family members. Psychoeducational multifamily groups teach families about the relationship between negative expressed emotion and relapse, train family members in skills to reduce their level of negative expressed emotion toward the patient, and help family members learn alternative means of coping and communicating (Dixon et al. 2001a).

Many studies consistently and overwhelmingly support the use of family psychoeducation in the treatment of schizophrenia. For example, individuals whose families participated in family psychoeducation experienced relapse and rehospitalization 40% less often than those who received individual therapy and medication alone. McFarlane's particular multifamily group format decreased the relapse rate by another 15% (Dixon et al. 2001a). Similar results have been shown for other problems. For example, substance abuse researchers found that teaching families of problem drinkers how to minimize their own distress and how to help increase the motivation of the substance-abusing family member resulted in more problem drinkers' seeking professional treatment and reducing their drinking even before they began treatment. Drinking was further reduced when family members were included in the substance abuse treatment (Sisson and Azrin 1986). Similar effects have been found with bipolar disorder. For example, in one recent study individuals with bipolar disorder were assigned either to family psychoeducation or to individual therapy, and participants in both groups were instructed to continue their normal medication routine. Patients in the family-focused treatment (psychoeducation) had fewer mood disorder relapses and were less likely to be rehospitalized than those in individual treatment (Rea et al. 2003).

With respect to psychoeducation in BPD, one study shows that, contrary to expectation, greater knowledge about BPD was associated with higher levels of burden, distress, and depression on the part of family members. These findings raise concerns both about the lack of standardized information about BPD and about the acquisition of information without the balancing effects of skills development (Hoffman et al. 2003a). Fortunately, at least two approaches to psychoeducation with BPD families seem to be helpful, although they are just beginning to be evaluated more fully.

John G. Gunderson developed a psychoeducation group, based on McFarlane's work with schizophrenia, for families of patients with BPD. His multifamily groups aim to increase patient functioning by decreasing negative expressed emotion within the family environment through education, support, and interpersonal skills training. Controlled trials have not yet been conducted, but preliminary data suggest that family members felt more supported, less burdened, and better able to communicate with their relative after participation in the group for 1 year.

● ● ●

An interesting study showed that families with a member who has BPD might be very different from families with a schizophrenic member in at least one important way: greater emotional involvement with the ill member seems beneficial in BPD families.

● ● ●

Perry D. Hoffman and Alan E. Fruzzetti developed a different approach to family psychoeducation based on ***dialectical behavior therapy (DBT),*** the very effective individual treatment for BPD (Linehan 1993). This approach to family psychoeducation, called DBT–family skills training (DBT-FST), has been offered both to groups of families and to individual families. The goal of treatment is twofold: 1) to enhance the success of the patient's individual treatment by teaching family members how to reinforce new behaviors the patient is learning in individual treatment, and 2) to improve the quality of the family environment for all its members. An interesting study showed that families with a member who has BPD might be very different from families with a schizophrenic member in at least one important way: greater emotional involvement with the ill member seems beneficial in BPD families (Hooley and Hoffman 1999). Therefore, DBT-FST programs take an approach that is substantially different from the more traditional psychoeducation groups noted above.

The first part of the 6-month DBT-FST program focuses on educating family members about the characteristics of BPD and their origins. The purpose of this portion of the program is to encourage understanding and empathy. Participants then learn how to become less judgmental of each other (and of themselves), reduce negative reactivity, and communicate more effectively by creating a mutually *validating* environment. Family members learn how they may have unknowingly discouraged effective behaviors and reinforced maladaptive patterns. To change these patterns, they are taught how to validate effective functioning in a consistent way. Individuals with BPD are taught how to reinforce effective interactions with their family members, thereby creating a partnership and a calmer, cooler home environment. The DBT-FST group provides a safe place to practice these new skills and have open discussions about intense issues (Hoffman et al. 1999). Preliminary results of multifamily psychoeducation show significant benefits for family members, such as reducing distress and increasing their reports of effective family communication. The program's benefits for the individuals with BPD have not been evaluated.

Some psychoeducational programs are meant to be used by consumers outside a treatment center and without the leadership of a therapist or other professional. *Bibliotherapy* is a term used to describe written self-help materials designed by professionals to be used by individuals on their own, but typically in conjunction with a professional consultation. This is not the same as simply purchasing self-help books at a bookstore, and little is known about the effectiveness of most self-help books. However, numerous controlled studies support the usefulness of bibliotherapy. For example, this approach is useful for decreasing harmful drinking in individuals seeking help for alcohol abuse. Self-help materials outlining specific strategies are more helpful than those offering general information and may be particularly useful for people who are unlikely to seek professional help because of stigma or denial of illness (Apodaca and Miller 2003). There are currently no studies of bibliotherapy for BPD, but given its success with other disorders and the lack of evidence-based treatments for BPD in many communities, this is a promising set of interventions in need of further research.

Concurrent Family Therapy

There are many different types of family therapy, and many different kinds of professionals (family therapists, psychiatrists, social workers, psychologists, and others) offer different versions of family therapy. This array of programs can be quite confusing for families seeking services. Fortunately, many of these programs—notably those focusing on improving relationships and interactions within the family—have been shown to be useful to families in general. Most importantly, many types of family therapy have been shown to help improve or augment the individual treatment (psychotherapy or medication) of a family member with a serious psychiatric disorder. For example, numerous studies show that couples therapy or family therapy can aid in the treatment of depression, bipolar disorder, schizophrenia, substance abuse, eating disorders, and a host of other problems.

Very few types of family therapy programs directed specifically to families of borderline patients have been evaluated. However, the lack of available evidence for the success of other types of family therapy in BPD does not mean that these treatments would not be useful in this disorder.

DBT has been shown to be effective in the individual treatment of both adults and adolescents with BPD. Building from the DBT model, DBT family therapy is a promising new approach to working with families with a member who has BPD (e.g., Fruzzetti and Fruzzetti 2003; Miller et al. 2002). These approaches to family therapy specify the treatment targets very clearly and focus explicitly on building skills within the family and improving family communication and interactions. Consequently, these approaches try to improve treatment outcomes for both the individual patient and other family members.

Family involvement in DBT may include engaging family members in a variety of activities, such as 1) learning about BPD, the DBT model for how the disorder develops, and how family interactions might be involved (in both positive and negative ways); 2) learning skills that the patient is also learning, both to help her or him (e.g., coaching) and to help the family member(s) deal with difficult or stressful situations; 3) learning how to change problematic cognitive, emotional, and verbal styles; 4) learning skills to change problematic patterns of family interaction; 5) learning effective communication skills; and 6) focusing on skills to enjoy relationships and activities in the family whenever possible.

Depending on the treatment setting, DBT with families may be offered to individual families, to multifamily groups with other families, to groups just for parents of adolescent or young adult patients, to groups just for couples or partners when the patient is an adult, or in other formats. Data show that these types of interventions may be very helpful to the patient in achieving her or his goals, as well as to family members who participate (A.E. Fruzzetti and J. Compton, unpublished manuscript, November 2004; Rathus and Miller 2002).

Researchers at the University of Iowa have developed a new treatment for BPD called Systems Training for Emotional Predictability and Problem Solving (STEPPS). Family members and significant others are an integral part of this treatment and are encouraged to attend educational sessions, where they are taught ways to support the treatment and reinforce newly acquired skills. There is not enough research yet to show that STEPPS is an effective treatment for BPD, but a preliminary study suggests that participation in STEPPS is associated with a moderate decrease in negative moods and impulsive behaviors (Blum et al. 2002).

Family Involvement to Improve Family Relationships and Family Functioning

There are dozens of different approaches to couples and family therapy designed to improve communication, problem solving, relationship satisfaction, and other aspects of family functioning. Fortunately, many of these approaches have been shown to work with a variety of families struggling with many kinds of difficulties. These therapies are often described as systemic (or systems) family therapy or as behavioral (or *cognitive-behavioral*) couple and family therapy, although there are many other varieties available. These types of family interventions in particular have accumulated extensive evidence showing that they work.

● ● ●

It is important for families to ask prospective family therapists about their experience with family functioning in BPD, the approach they will use, and the evidence for its effectiveness.

● ● ●

Family therapy can be of either short duration (just a few visits) or long duration (lasting a year or more) and typically involves having all involved family members present if possible. Treatment may focus on describing problems; trying new methods of discussing problems or difficulties; building skills; uncovering the motivation, meaning, or function of problem behaviors that were poorly understood in the past; activating or reactivating strengths already existing in family relationships; and a variety of other activities. Homework or practice between sessions is common.

Because there has been relatively little research on family therapy with families who have a member with BPD, it is important for families to ask prospective family therapists about their experience with family functioning in BPD. Some questions family members may find useful to ask before making a commitment to therapy include the following: What kind of therapy does the therapist practice? What kind of approach will be used? What evidence exists for the effectiveness of that approach? Fortunately, more research is exploring the needs of families that must deal with BPD; as a result, more specific and effective treatments will evolve and therapists will be more attuned to the questions families ask in their search for family therapy that meets their needs.

Family Involvement to Reduce Family Stress and Burden

Much of the research on family interventions (family psychoeducation and family therapy) has focused on improving patient outcomes. Although most treatments involving family members recognize the importance of family well-being to successful patient outcomes, the primary goal of family treatment is most often to reduce symptoms and improve functioning in the individual with BPD. However, several programs have been developed just for family members, specifically to reduce the stress and burden of caring for a family member with a severe psychiatric disorder.

Programs primarily targeting family well-being, often called family support or family education programs, differ from family psychoeducation in several notable ways (Solomon 1996). For example, family education groups tend to be led by trained volunteers (who are usually family members of patients themselves) rather than by professionals. These kinds of programs are often based in the community rather than in hospitals or clinics. Thus they are not technically considered treatment, but rather programs offering education and the support of others affected by the disorder. The grassroots nature of these programs and the voluntary status of the their leaders allows many to offer participation in groups free of charge or for very minimal fees.

Many family education and support programs were originally developed for caregivers of persons with severe, chronic medical conditions. For example, an analysis of 78 studies of different kinds of interventions with families of Alzheimer's disease patients showed that psychoeducational and skills-oriented family treatments had the most consistent and significant positive effects on family members' well-being. Participants in these programs consistently reported decreased depression and sense of burden and increases in overall well-being, knowledge of the illness, and ability to take care of their family member (Sörensen et al. 2002).

The National Alliance for the Mentally Ill (NAMI) offers a free 12-week family education course, called Family-to-Family, for families with a member who has severe mental illness. The goals of the course are to decrease the stigma, isolation, and hopelessness of family members through education and empathic understanding. NAMI courses are led by trained family members who provide information about mental illness and rehabilitation and who train participants in self-care, communication, and problem-solving skills. Unlike formal family psychoeducation programs, the course is not diagnosis specific, but it does tend to focus on schizophrenia, bipolar disorder, depression, obsessive-compulsive disorder, and panic disorder. An uncontrolled pilot study found that course participants felt significantly less displeasure and worry about their ill family members and felt more empowered within their families, communities, and relatives' treatment teams. Furthermore, these improvements were maintained 6 months after the course ended (Dixon et al. 2001b).

The National Education Alliance for Borderline Personality Disorder (NEA-BPD) offers a free 12-week program for family members of persons with BPD, called Family CONNECTIONS. This course—based on theories and skills from both DBT for individuals and DBT with couples and families—was developed using feedback from family members and consumers. The course is led by trained family members, who follow a structured and tested curriculum and provide participants with the most current information about BPD and the opportunity to build a support network while learning new skills. Initial research shows that Family CONNECTIONS is very beneficial to family members. For example, participants report significantly lower levels of depression, grief, and burden and increases in mastery and self-concept after participation in the program (Hoffman et al. 2003b).

Conclusion

There is a long history of family involvement in treatment (psychoeducation or family therapy) resulting in significant treatment gains for individuals with severe disorders. Similarly, family treatments have been shown to help ameliorate problems in families more generally. Despite the relatively small number of studies of programs designed for families with a member with BPD, several programs have been shown to be helpful. In addition, family member–led groups for parents or partners of BPD patients have shown promise in alleviating individual distress and depression among family caregivers. With the new energy emerging in the past few years, it is likely that the coming decade will bring new programs and evidence to provide relief for individuals with BPD and their loved ones.

What Families Need to Know

Key Messages in This Chapter

- Involving the family in the treatment of serious psychiatric problems has been shown to be beneficial to both patients and family members.
- When choosing a treatment program for BPD (or any other psychiatric disorder), it is essential for consumers and their families to have information about the effectiveness of that particular treatment.
- Family psychoeducation builds on a family's strengths and does not blame the family for the patient's difficulties.
- There is strong evidence for the effectiveness of family psychoeducation programs in improving symptoms in individuals with schizophrenia, bipolar disorder, and alcohol abuse.
- Several forms of psychoeducation have been adapted specifically for patients and families with BPD. One such program incorporates the principles of dialectical behavior therapy (DBT); it helps families learn the skills that will enhance their loved one's individual treatment program.
- DBT family therapy is a promising new approach that uses the principles of DBT to build communication skills and improve interaction within the family.
- Family support or family education programs, usually led by volunteer family members, offer families current information and mutual support, as well as training in problem solving and self-care. The Family CONNECTIONS course, developed specifically for family members of individuals with BPD, has been shown to provide them with some relief from the burden of caring for their family member with BPD.

Key Words in This Chapter

bibliotherapy   the use of written self-help materials designed to be used under the direction of a professional.

case studies or case reports   reports describing a particular patient or treatment.

cognitive-behavioral therapies   therapies focusing on thoughts, feelings, and actions the person is aware of; treatment is aimed at using the thinking process to reframe, restructure, and solve problems.

dialectical behavior therapy (DBT)   a treatment for BPD developed by Marsha Linehan combining aspects of cognitive and behavioral therapy. The treatment teaches specific skills to manage emotions, control impulsiveness, and diminish self-destructive behavior.

expressed emotion   a concept measuring the attitudes and beliefs of family members toward their relative with a mental illness.

family therapy   treatment typically involving all members of the family, with a focus on improving relationships and interactions within the family.

psychoeducation   programs that provide illness-specific information and coping strategies, with the aim of improving patient functioning and reducing the burden on the family.

randomized controlled trials   studies in which subjects are assigned randomly to treatment or control groups to determine whether the treatment being studied is effective.

validation, validating   legitimizing the emotions, thoughts, and experiences of another.

How to Find Out About Resources Locally, Nationally, and Internationally

National Education Alliance for Borderline Personality Disorder (NEA-BPD)
Family CONNECTIONS
P.O. Box 974
Rye, NY 10580
Phone: (914) 835-9011
E-mail: NEABPD@aol.com
http://www.borderlinepersonalitydisorder.com

Borderline Personality Disorder Resource Center
Macy Villa, New York-Presbyterian Hospital, Westchester Division
21 Bloomingdale Road
White Plains, NY 10605
Phone: (914) 682-5496; (888) 694-2273
E-mail: info@bpdresourcecenter.org
http://bpdresourcecenter.org

References

Apodaca T, Miller W: A meta-analysis of the effectiveness of bibliotherapy for alcohol problems. J Clin Psychol 59:289–304, 2003

Blum N, Pfohl B, St. John D, et al: STEPPS: a cognitive-behavioral systems-based group treatment for outpatients with borderline personality disorder—a preliminary report. Compr Psychiatry 43:301–310, 2002

Dixon L, McFarlane WR, Lefley H, et al: Evidence-based practices for services to families of people with psychiatric disabilities. Psychiatr Serv 52:903–910, 2001a

Dixon L, Stewart B, Burland J, et al: Pilot study on the effectiveness of the family-to-family education program. Psychiatr Serv 52:965–967, 2001b

Fruzzetti AE, Fruzzetti AR: Borderline personality disorder: dialectical behavior therapy with couples, in Treating Difficult Couples: Helping Clients With Coexisting Mental and Relationship Disorders. Edited by Snyder D, Whisman MA. New York, Guilford, 2003, pp 235–260

Hoffman PD, Fruzzetti AE, Swenson CR: Dialectical behavior therapy—family skills training. Fam Process 38:399–414, 1999

Hoffman PD, Buteau E, Hooley JM, et al: Family members' knowledge about borderline personality disorder: correspondence with their levels of depression, burden, distress, and expressed emotion. Fam Process 42:469–478, 2003a

Hoffman PD, Fruzzetti AE, Buteau E, et al: Family connections: a dialectical support and educational approach for families of persons with borderline personality disorder. Paper presented at the meeting of the International Society for the Investigation and Teaching of Dialectical Behavior Therapy, Boston, MA, November 2003b

Hooley JM, Hoffman PD: Expressed emotion and clinical outcome in borderline personality disorder. Am J Psychiatry 156:1557–1562, 1999

Linehan MM: Cognitive-Behavioral Treatment of Borderline Personality Disorder. New York, Guilford, 1993

McFarlane WR, Dixon L, Lukens E, et al: Family psychoeducation and schizophrenia: a review of the literature. J Marital Fam Ther 29:223–245, 2003

Miller AL, Glinski J, Woodberry K, et al: Family therapy and dialectical behavior therapy with adolescents: part 1, proposing a clinical synthesis. Am J Psychother 56:568–584, 2002

Rathus JH, Miller AL: Dialectical behavior therapy adapted for suicidal adolescents. Suicide Life Threat Behav 32:146–157, 2002

Rea MM, Tompson MC, Miklowitz DJ, et al: Family-focused treatment versus individual treatment for bipolar disorder: results of a randomized clinical trial. J Consult Clin Psychol 71:482–492, 2003

Sisson RW, Azrin NH: Family members' involvement to initiate and promote the treatment of problem drinkers. J Behav Ther Exp Psychiatry 17:15–21, 1986

Solomon P: Moving from psychoeducation to family education for families of adults with serious mental illness. Psychiatr Serv 47:1364–1370, 1996

Sörensen S, Pinquart M, Duberstein P: How effective are interventions with caregivers? An updated meta-analysis. Gerontologist 42:356–372, 2002

Index

*Page numbers printed in **boldface** type refer to tables.*